... own kind

...magine a book written in such

...es would ...ve a hazy quality, but in fact its clarity of expression is startling. It's a fireworks display. It's also a profound meditation on language and loss and time, and on how we construct ourselves through stories. And it's painful. And it's beautiful. And I love it. Samantha Harvey is the most exceptionally gifted of authors, and here she demonstrates that she can literally do anything'

Nathan Filer

'It's a claustrophobic, enlightening, moving, existential treatise on sleep, insomnia and death. And it's funny, too'

Guardian

'I am still shuddering, almost, from the beautiful, beautiful writing and its broken, angry, vibrant demand – a dare almost – to accept life, and brave it, with all it brings' Cynan Jones

'A creative account of a life with little sleep... Readers looking for their own cure will instead find an erudite companion to help them through the dark times'

Sunday Times

'It's funny, sad, wry, always worrying away at the mystery of sleep and its absence and finding endless new angles so that the whole has something of the quality of those waking dreams that haunt the insomniac and are her private country'

SAMANTHA HARVEY

Samantha Harvey is the author of *The Wilderness*, *All Is Song*, *Dear Thief*, and *The Western Wind*. She appeared on the longlists for the Bailey's Prize and the Man Booker, and the shortlists of the James Tait Black Award, the Orange Prize, the Guardian First Book Award and the Walter Scott Prize. *The Wilderness* won the Betty Trask Award in 2009. She is a tutor on the MA course in Creative Writing at Bath Spa University.

ALSO BY SAMANTHA HARVEY

The Wilderness
All Is Song
Dear Thief
The Western Wind

SAMANTHA HARVEY

The Shapeless Unease

VINTAGE

1 3 5 7 9 10 8 6 4 2

Vintage
20 Vauxhall Bridge Road,
London SW1V 2SA

Vintage is part of the Penguin Random House group of companies
whose addresses can be found at global.penguinrandomhouse.com

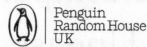 Penguin
Random House
UK

First published in the UK by Jonathan Cape in 2020
First published by Vintage in 2021

penguin.co.uk/vintage

A CIP catalogue record for this book is available
from the British Library

ISBN 9781529112092

Printed and bound in Great Britain by Clays Ltd, Elcograf S.p.A.

Penguin Random House is committed to a sustainable future
for our business, our readers and our planet. This book is
made from Forest Stewardship Council® certified paper.

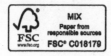

MIX
Paper from
responsible sources
FSC
www.fsc.org   FSC® C018179

For all those awake in the night.

And for those I've woken up; I'm sorry.

Friend: What are you writing?

Me: Not sure, some essays. Not really essays. Not essays at all. Some things.

Friend: About what?

Me: Not sure. This and that. About not sleeping, mainly. But death keeps creeping in.

Friend: Murgh.

Me: Murgh what?

Friend: Murgh morbid.

Me: But we're all going to—

Friend: But we're not yet.

Me: But we are, every day.

Friend: We're living every day.

Me: In the midst of life we are in—

Friend: Pff.

Me: In the midst of life we are—

Friend: Why don't you write another novel instead?

Me: My cousin died, alone in his flat. They think
           he'd been dead for two days by the time they
           found him. He wasn't very old.

Friend: Oh.

Me: It's not – I just – we weren't even that close.

Friend: Rotten.

Me: I can't stop thinking of him in his coffin in the
           ground.

Friend: And yet, best not to.

Me: When I think about it, grief wells up in me so
           large, pure grief, as if for all the people I'm go-
           ing to lose. As if his death is a doorway into all
           deaths. What stops the parasitoid wasps and
           predatory beetles eating my mother's eyes? I'm
           a child being hushed to sleep by her or eating
           pilchards on toast with her or reading Roald
           Dahl with her or walking with her to school or
           being sponged down by her while I burn with
           hives, and now I imagine that she is having her
           organs eaten by her gut bacteria and she's
           decaying. And I can't breathe, for the grief I feel.

           My cousin's death has invited all deaths.

           I can't breathe with this future grief.

Friend: [Has gone.]

∞

Midnight:

Into bed and lie down. Head goes on pillow.

Out of bed; superstitiously plucking the strewn clothes from the floor to fold them into rough bundles and put them away – one of countless little routines undertaken to forfend a sleepless night. One of countless little routines forcibly dismissed as superstition, in the superstition that superstitious acts will only shorten the odds of sleep – but unignorable in the end. Needs must. The attaining of sleep long ago left the realm of natural act and entered that of black magic.

Back into bed and read, a collection of William Trevor short stories. There's sleepiness soon, like something calling from around the corner. There's a sharp, stinging pain at the crown of my head; the scalp is being stitched with embroidery needles. The lamp is shut off and the room is more or less dark. An odd creak issues from who knows where.

The heart starts up its thrup-thrup-thrup, a tripping percussion in a chest that now fills with breath. Breathe, breathe. And with the light out, here they come, all of them, the holy and the horrifying; here they are.

In the medieval *Ars moriendi* the deathbed of a man is crowded with them, saints and demons, each vying for his soul. The demons try to tempt him into despair – there's something monkey-like with horns and a man's face on its belly, holding a dagger; something dog-like with a single antler and a perverse grin, a luring finger; a ram-headed demon looking over his shoulder; a satyr-like being with a hooked nose, licking its lips. Come with us into death, they say. Forsake your faith and come with us.

And then a picture of the same man, the satyr fallen at his bedside, the leg of another demon that has scrambled in fear under the bed. Mary Magdalene and St Peter stand by his pillow, St Peter holding the key to heaven. Behind them, Jesus is crucified, his head slumped backwards over the horizontal strut of the cross, and on the headboard of the bed is the rooster of Peter's redemption, the rooster whose crow awoke him from his denial of Christ and caused him to repent. Come with us, say the rooster, St Peter, the Christ – here is your restoration, come with us to the kingdom of heaven.

I close my eyes and try to keep hold of that sleepiness, whose call is still there behind the heart's syncopation. The heart a tough lump of meat, flooded with fear. Fifty minutes pass; it's almost one. Usually if sleep is going to come it would have come by now; and if it hasn't come by now, the probability is no sleep at all. Sweat, the first inkling of panic like a storm heard across a distant plain, just the vaguest muffled thunder. Still time to sleep; the storm might yet not come.

St Peter hovers with the key; take it, he says, it'll get you there. I reach out and the Devil steps in – because the desire for sleep is also the denial of it; the more you want it the less it comes. The word *greed* is whispered somewhere from the darkness. *You are too greedy for sleep.* Jesus slumps backwards, dead, mouth agape at the ceiling. The word *come* is whispered afterwards and I don't know from which quarter. Saint or demon? I don't know.

Have faith, I hear. Have hope.

Lose faith, I hear. Give up hope.

Heart thrup-thrup-thrup, scalp tight. Now my small room is over-brimming. The louder thrupping of my heart. The churning of the air. The wingbeats of the harpy, claws out, cheeks sunken in hunger, Peter sidling up towards my pillow.

Lying on one side, cradling my head. Sleepiness vanishes, like the picture when you turned off an old TV screen; it recedes to a dot. Then there's blankness and blackness; the yawning expanse of a night awake.

∞

My cousin's next to us in the church in a sealed box, with his skin buffed to a plausible pallor and his eyes and lips

5

glued shut. His arteries, once livid with blood, are now sluggish with embalming fluid, and his out-of-sight orifices plugged. His body running with stitches from a post-mortem. Skull cut open with a hand-saw and re-sewn, organs removed and approximately replaced – heart a bit far to the left, lungs a bit lopsided (hard to put them back how they were), tongue and windpipe missing. Hair washed and brushed. Shirt buttoned.

On his chest, Michael Palin's *Pole to Pole* and *Himalaya*.

To my right, my aunt wailing quietly through a closed mouth, the sound you might make involuntarily if somebody sat on your chest.

When he was born, my cousin, it was with a facial deformity, a lump whose removal left his cheek badly scarred, but scarred in a way that stopped being visible to those of us who knew him. Over the years the scar became gentle and weathered. Ill-luck was his birthright, this deforming lump and then epilepsy, seizures both regular and severe. But he'd run at his unlucky life with a quiet verve; he travelled a long way in his short time on this earth. He went to places far-flung, and usually alone. He loved Byron Bay, he took his bike to Australia and only then realised (how only then?) that it was too big to cycle around.

Thailand, Indonesia, Myanmar, Singapore, Canada, Mozambique, Russia, Mexico, Cuba, Brazil, Japan, most of Europe (I'm making it up, I don't remember the eulogy's list, was too busy eyeing the coffin to my right and thinking, *he is in there, dead*). A spare weekend came, or a week off work, and he'd get on a flight somewhere, or he'd get on his bike and go for hours, and one Saturday when I was doing a signing at a bookshop in Rye, not far from where he lived, he said he'd cycle down and see me; he wrote afterwards to say he was sorry he didn't come, he couldn't make it. That was the last time we had contact with one another. My uncle texted him a joke the day after he died, and worried when he didn't get a reply, and I often wonder if there is a sadder thing in all the world than that unread joke on a dead person's phone. A Facebook post shows the mapped route of a seventy-mile bike ride he did alone on what was probably the day he died. At the funeral I saw him as a child in our nan's garden by the low wall, and I saw his widest of smiles, and I saw him dead in his bed – not face down, as he was found, but face up, with his grafted skin faintly puckering a cheek that had smashed god knows how many times against a kitchen floor or chair leg.

Epilepsy could kill him at any time – if his head thrashed against tarmac, or the enamel of a bath, or if he was cycling, or if he swallowed his tongue, or if he had a fit and never came round.

What is it to be so close to death so often? Yet he dodged it all those times.

Yet it caught him that once, and with death that's all it takes.

∞

Case study of possible chronic Post Brexit Insomnia (PBI):

Patient, female, forty-three, has always slept well. She reports both ease of going to sleep and of staying asleep, usually for around eight hours a night. This pattern has tended to hold even in times of stress and difficulty.

The patient reports that her problems with sleep began a few months after she moved house to live on a main road, when she was often woken early by traffic. This happened for several months and resulted in her sleep being disturbed. She states that she was not, at this point, an insomniac, only suffering somewhat disturbed sleep.

Over a period of months, her sleep disturbances fluctuated. In June 2016 they began to be accompanied by anger at the result of the European Referendum, resulting in periods of restless wakefulness. By the autumn of this year she was not only waking up early with the traffic, but finding it difficult to go to sleep at bedtime.

During this period she battled with anger and frustration at both the traffic and at the unfolding senselessness of politics, and found herself 'arguing' (patient's expression) with the passing cars, lorries, vans and buses. She knew that there was no point in arguing in this way, and tried various strategies for endurance (earplugs, white-noise generation, alcohol slightly exceeding the recommended upper range), as well as for acceptance (mindfulness meditation, Buddhist mantras, affirmations of loving-kindness), but found them of limited use, and reports unbidden fantasies of multi-car pile-ups, earthquakes and freak cosmic events which might lead to the temporary or permanent closure of the road.

By October of the year in question, her sleep problems had become what she would now call insomnia – difficulty going to sleep and staying asleep. She went on a silent Buddhist retreat and reports great comfort in the sound of the wind hitting her window and the pervasion of quiet, but did not find any improvement in her sleep. Indeed, it was here that she first detected the existence of persistent panic, even when engaged in easeful and calm activities.

On arriving home from the retreat, she recalls meeting her next-door neighbour at the bus stop, who told her of the death of their lodger; this was a man not much known by the patient, but she had seen him putting the bins out only the week before, and the sadness for his death, though without lasting impact, was real and 'a reminder of how quickly people are snatched from us'. Later that day she was informed of the separation of her sister and partner, and reports feelings of shock and sadness, for both her sister and partner, and for their three young children. Some days after this, she learned of the death of her cousin, who was found in his flat two days after he passed away. Some days later she was informed that her father's partner had been diagnosed with dementia. A week or two after her cousin's funeral, she learned that her father had fallen from a ladder, had badly broken his leg and would be unable to walk for a year.[1]

Her sleep problems worsened over the coming weeks. Though there was some unaccounted-for respite from insomnia during December of that year, it returned in January and continued from there to worsen steadily. She reports many nights of two or three hours of sleep, these hours not always consecutive, and nights of zero sleep. In this time she tried sleeping in other rooms of the house, and moved her desk from her study to create

---

[1] Question these factors as sufficient triggers for insomnia? Deaths not those of people intimate to her. Note patient has been prone in recent past to psychosomatic disorders and Over-reactive Disorder (OD).

a makeshift bedroom. This gave respite from noise, but no recovery of sleep. Sleeping aids – over-the-counter (Nytol, Sominex, Dormeasan drops, CBD oil, magnesium powders, passion flower, hop strobiles, melatonin, 5HTP) and prescription (Zopiclone, Diazepam, Mirtazapine) – were of little use.

The patient tried many remedial approaches, including visits to a CBT sleep clinic, acupuncture, a stress-reduction mindfulness course, sleep restriction techniques, gratitude diaries, dietary supplements, abstention from caffeine and sugar, and a sleep device that emits alpha, beta and theta waves to mimic the stages of sleep. Her approaches also included experimenting with bedtimes and finding ways to occupy and calm herself during her hours of wakefulness. She reports learning French, making mosaics, playing solitaire, doing jigsaws, counting her breaths, listening to episodes of *In Our Time*, Tate podcasts, *The Allusionist*, an audio edition of *Remembrance of Things Past*, Radio 4's *Soul Music*, online sleep hypnosis meditations, a birdsong identification CD, episodes of *Poldark* and *The Crown*, Sanskrit chanting and *Top of the Pops*.[2]

She reports that her aim shifted from trying to sleep to trying not to panic, and that some nights she would lie

***

[2] Consider *Top of the Pops* as aggravating factor?

in darkness for seven hours, counting backwards from one thousand in threes, or counting backwards from one hundred in French or German, or chanting along to the Sanskrit, which she knew only as sounds rather than as words, but onto which she imposed peaceful meanings, and which she found soothing.

Her abiding feelings over these weeks and months were of anger, loneliness, despair and fear. She suffered recurring images of her cousin in his coffin underground, images accompanied by palpitations and panic. Death occupied many of her thoughts, along with a concern – prompted by a dream – that the journey into death would be fearful and lonely, a 'hellish hurtle in a dark shuttle'. She was disturbed by the thought of her cousin suffering this journey, and also began to project the deaths of her loved ones.[3] She also reports suspicions of having Fatal Familial Insomnia, an extremely rare hereditary disease resulting in premature death.[4]

---

[3] See Fleming, Feldman et al., 'Proliferation of Pointless Mortality Projection Syndrome (PMPS): a clinico-pathological study of thanatophobia and mental health disorders'.

[4] Note: new manifestation of OD? Consider that patient's fear of illness and death presents as a contradictory *willing* of illness and death through constant imagination.

In the night she found herself re-experiencing certain memories from childhood, not so much as memories but as events being lived, such as her mother leaving and her dog dying, and these recollections brought grief and rage. She likened this to the grief and rage she felt in response to the loss – through the result of the Referendum – of many of the values she had once attached to her country, and which had given her a sense of national belonging, pride and identification.[5]

The panic she had detected at the retreat the previous autumn was by now resulting in fierce attacks at night, during which she would hyperventilate, convulse and hit her head, either with her own fists or against a wall. She reports that this behaviour was the result of increasingly severe sleep deprivation.

The patient's work and social life became unviable during these months; she could no longer work in a sustained or coherent way. She saw little of her friends and relied heavily upon the support of her partner. By now she was experiencing around three or four nights a week of no sleep, and intermittent sleep the remaining nights. She would regularly stay awake for forty or fifty hours.

[5] Refer to Smith, Carroll, Walsh et al., 'Post Brexit Insomnia: the effect of direct democracy on circadian function and the thalamus'.

Physical symptoms of sleeplessness included confusion, memory loss, palpitations, severe headaches, hair loss, eye infections and numbness in her hands.

She claims that she awaited a breakdown and that this breakdown would be welcome. She believed that if the issue, which eluded her, could come to a head, she might then be left broken, but broken free of it. At the same time she very much doubted she would have a breakdown, surmising that there wasn't anything decisive enough in her character to bring one about, and that she was more the kind of person who would endure pain and suffering indefinitely while just about managing to cope.

This feeling, she reports, was reinforced by the fact that, at night, she felt increasingly feral, like a wild animal enduring a cage, and would pace, make sounds of obvious distress and pull at her hair, behaviour that didn't seem to come from her conscious being, but from a wild part of herself below or beyond consciousness. Yet by day, although exhausted and subdued, she continued to function at a relatively normal – if much reduced – capacity, with intact levels of reason and perspective, much reduced (although not no) anger, and no desire to hit her head or cause any harm to herself or others.

She reports that she did not understand where the wildness came from at night, nor where it went by day. She reports being terrified of it, yet at times wishing for it to take over, and describes powerful, yearning imaginings of being admitted to hospital and drugged, or of having suffered a complete and debilitating breakdown and being surrounded by loved ones. In this scene she reports that she cannot see herself at all, so surrounded she is by those carers, and nor does she have any autonomy, needs or wishes, so subsumed is her being, she says, by the overwhelming force of their care.

∞

Dear Cousin Paul,

I write without flippancy. I write to tell you what Google tells me you should expect from your first days, weeks and months of death. I write to try to guard you from disappointments surrounding your fate. I wish only that you could write back.

A corpse in a coffin underground will take half a century to rot down to dust (good news? I felt this was somewhat good news). The femur so relied upon by you until a few days ago, when you went for that bike ride, will fight the good fight underground and resist the dissolution of its lovely tree-trunk shaft, its gentle rooted knee-splay; it'll hold on to its subtle curve even when the marrow is shot and the bone snappable. With nothing to snap it, it'll lie in blackness like a fading X-ray, disintegrating, yes, of course disintegrating, but still there, the persistence of your material being. For a whole fifty years.

Yet – your face. Your face with the scar tissue spread across your cheek; that little bit where your upper lip folds in a tiny neatness to form the bridge between nostrils, and that nice thing that happens when you look up suddenly, in curiosity, and years blur and you look like you did when you were a child. Your face and its billion moments of life will collapse and rot, and within a few weeks the corpse will be hard to recognise as you.

Even before you were buried your organs will have started to decay; almost straight away that'll have happened, when you were still on your bed, during those days before you were found. *Autolysis*: self-digestion. The bacteria in your gut will have begun to eat dead cells, and a greenish stain will have appeared on your abdomen. Then these bacteria spread to the stomach, to the chest, the thighs, the legs—

What an unlikely wonder is life, that it holds in itself the whole wildness of death – those bacteria didn't come into life at the point of death, they were always there and they always wanted to eat you, and your cells always contained in them the enzymes that would assist your rotting. It was only ever your vehemence to survive that prevented all that. Did you know, were you ever able to detect within, the passionate warfare that kept you here?

And then the war is fought and finished, and the process of unexisting you begins. Bacteria swarm through you, and as they digest you they let off gases that make you rise like dough, and on your third or fourth day of death you're beginning to smell, and you're a vibrant, moving mass of activity. Methane, odours, swelling, morphing, the escaping of your tongue from your mouth, fluids through your nose, your intestines through your rectum, a blooming, a slow-motion explosion, the busyness of life's oldest, most efficient and venerable clean-up operation.

What improbable teamwork, a tireless, Disney-like vigour. Vish-vash-vosh, aye-oh, aye-oh, the optimism and synchronicity of a midget army, a dash of vanishing-dust, a choral song of death, a transformation, and Bibbidi-Bobbidi-Boo, lo-and-behold, the fingers that had not long been blue begin a creeping shift to something blacker, and the explosion ceases with the same slow order in which it began, and the gases are ebbing, and the body collapses, a climax reached, a slackening of flesh, the first troops withdraw, we are here at the next stage after only fifteen or so days of death if we're not yet embalmed: *black putrefaction*. The flesh turns creamy against patches of bruising, the body lies in a pool of fluid, the predatory beetles come, the maggots, the parasitoid wasps—

But you're embalmed, so, fifteen days in, this isn't happening to you. My dear cousin, not yet. You're safe in the eternal night of your coffin, away from (unable ever to return to) everyone you ever loved, with your skull sawn in half.

Cousin Paul, cousin Paul.

At the bottom of the webpage that's telling me all this about your inevitable descent into black putrefaction, it says:

> *If you are struggling, consider online therapy with BetterHelp.*
>
> *You are worth it!*

∞

'Let me explain about the sleep cycle. Do you know about the sleep cycle?'

'Not really.'

'I'll draw a diagram.'

'I just feel so—'

'Anxious.'

'And angry.'

'Anger is no use when we want to sleep.'

'I know.'

'Let's say this circle represents a full sleep cycle. The whole cycle takes about ninety minutes and a good sleeper will have around five of these cycles a night. This segment here is called Stage 1, and it's what we call light sleep – then comes Stage 2, which we call intermediate sleep. Making sense? Now, overall, this is the longest stage and most of the night will be spent here. It's very restful and this sleep is nice and refreshing for the body, but it isn't the most restorative phase. The most restorative is Stage 3, deep sleep. When you're in this phase your heart rate falls and you won't wake up unless something or somebody disturbs you, and even then it will be difficult to wake you. In the first two or so sleep cycles this stage will last around half an hour, but with each cycle it becomes shorter, so that you spend less time there. All OK so far? Then comes this stage, which we call REM sleep, Stage 4. This is where we dream, and it's kind of opposite to the deep-sleep phase. Our heart rate quickens, and with each cycle this phase gets longer. At first it's just ten minutes or so, but in the last one or two cycles it'll last around half an hour. Then we're all the way back round to Stage 1 again – light sleep, almost awake. We might wake up in this stage, in the middle of the night. We often do. That's natural and normal even for a good sleeper. And then the cycle begins again.'

'_'

'We want to get you having some nice, full sleep cycles, and a bit more of that deep-sleep phase.'

'The thing is, there's so much that's not right, so much suffering. My sister, my dad, my stepmum, I want to support them but I'm so knackered from not sleeping, I can barely function. I worry. About everything. About my family, about not sleeping. I've stopped writing. I go in to the university and teach with zero hours' sleep, I sit there and start a sentence and have no idea what word will come next or how I'll find my way to the end of it. I can feel my skin. It's too tight.'

'Is lack of sleep affecting your mental health, would you say?'

'I'm desperate, I want to know that it's going to end. I want to be there for my family. I could cope with it if I knew it would end, if somebody could reassure me.'

'I'm not going to reassure you. This isn't about a sticking plaster, this is about helping you change your behaviour and your thoughts.'

'I don't know what's wrong with my behaviour and thoughts.'

'That's what we're here to find out.'

'I never needed to have the right thought before, I slept, I didn't need special sleeping thoughts.'

'You need to believe that you can sleep again.'

'Since when was sleep a matter of faith?'

'You need to try to change your negativity into positivity.'

'I just want to be reassured.'

'We can easily get stuck in a "yes, but" pattern. Whenever help is offered, the response is "yes, but". It's about moving away from that. Having a "yes" mentality, not a "yes, but" one.'

'Yes.'

∞

But – you try having a positive mental attitude when you've had five hours' sleep in three nights. You try.

I lie in bed repeating the word for hours. Yesyesyesyes
yesyesyesyesyesyesyesyesyesyesyesyesyesyesyesyesyesyes
yesyesyesyesyesyes.

What does Y E S spell?

Yes.

What does E Y E S spell?

E-yes.

Yesyesyesyesyesyesyesyesyesyesyesyes.

Eyeseyeseyeseyeseyeseyeseyeseyeseyes.

Yesyesyesyesyesyesyesyesyesyes.

Eyeseyeseyeseyeseyeseyeseyeseyeseyes.

Closeyoureyescloseyoureyescloseyoureyesclose
youreyes.

Close you're yes.

Close you are, yes.

Yes.

Yes?

∞

Dust and ashes though I am, I sleep the sleep of angels.

This is the first line of my most recently published
novel. I don't know the person who wrote that line. The
person who wrote it didn't know anything. She didn't
know the first thing about anything.

Dust and ashes though I am are not even her words; they are the first words of St Augustine's *Confessions of a Sinner. I sleep the sleep of angels* are her words, but she knows nothing of angels and knew nothing then about sleep (in the way fish know nothing about water), she was just hazarding guesses, she was as green as a shoot.

But my sleep was ragged that night, she wrote. But she didn't know anything about ragged sleep when she wrote that. She knew the word *ragged* and she knew it was an adjective that could describe many things, including sleep, but she knew nothing about ragged sleep. Nowadays she is shocked by the fraudulence of words. Every word claims an authority and every word craves to be believed, and we read others' words and we find something to relate to, solace in a shared experience. Yet there doesn't have to be any experience behind a word. A word can be a shadow not cast by any object.

Lately, whenever I read that someone in a novel is having trouble sleeping my heart lurches forward to unite first with them, and then with their author, as if the ability to write the words guarantees a knowledge of the words written. Yet a word is just a collection of letters attached to an idea. The idea doesn't have to be attached to anything in the world. You can be rich in words and poor in experience, and you can spend, spend, spend, and somehow make that your living.

My sleep was ragged that night, wrote our little fraudster. Much is said to disparage authors who write outside of their expertise, and worse still, who appropriate the experience of others about whom they cannot know – a white man appropriating the experience of a Bangladeshi woman, a childless woman that of a mother – but nobody took the pen from my hand when I, well-slept, found a notion in my brain of sleeplessness. To write fiction you have to engage in organised fraud, the laundering of experience into the offshore haven of words.

Our little fraudster had a thousand more words than she had experiences; she was compelled to lie. Believe nothing she says. A word can be a little piece of inheritance. It can be spent without ever having been earned.

∞

1 a.m.:

Lie here then. Just lie here. What of it? It's just lying here. Think of good things.

The sky in France – so vast, so black, so star-spangled that when we got out of the car our gazes were pulled up to it, both of us at once, and we stood silently gaping. The Milky Way was a wide, distinct bow flexed above us and the stars – staggering in their numbers – did in fact twinkle.

The sunsets in France, a roaring red horizon and the hazy moon above, like a moth smoked out of a fire; Venus, Mars, Jupiter and Saturn all visible at once. Bats pouring out of the ruined tower of the medieval chateau, swooping above our heads and pouring in again. The fading call of crickets. My swimming costume hanging on the balcony railings going loose with chlorine and overuse, loose with two months of swimming.

I think about the swimming. I have a shell brought back for me from Oman, a conch that is smooth and white and fits well in the palm, and I've taken to holding it at night. Every now and then I'll let go of it long enough for it to become cold again. Think about the swimming, going up and down the pool following the lining seam. My underwater slipstream, my hands ageless and bright. Count your blessings. Lying here, thinking of the sunsets and swimming and the planets and stars, what is there to be afraid of? Try to calm the banging heart.

There's something called 'nocturnal forgiveness', which is the act of letting go of all wrongs and all guilt or blame, just for the duration of the night. You leave them outside the room. I forgive everything I can think of one by one – the cars driving past too fast, the jackdaws for ransacking the bird feeder, the universe for torturing me, myself for torturing me. What I suddenly think of is my dad plaiting my hair when I was nine years old, in the first few weeks after my mum left. Plaiting my hair with his huge, scarred, leathery builder's hands.

It's half past one, quarter to two. I'm trying to collect plums that have fallen from a tree onto the floor of a restaurant, burgundy plums, very ripe, some trodden in. Simultaneous to this comes the knowledge that I must be dreaming and therefore partly asleep, and with the realisation of this I have the swiftest moment of triumph – I'm asleep! – before waking up.

I don't look at a clock in the night but I've spent so many nights awake that I usually know the time within around ten or twenty minutes; I know the texture of the passing hours and the texture of my thoughts as the night abrades them. Around now they begin to show signs of wear. The little calm persuasions become frustrations. The forgiveness becomes laughable, and all the forgiven things that should be outside the room are in fact hovering about by my bed half-satisfied as if there's something else they need from me.

I want to go back to that dream of the plums. I open my eyes wide and close them in the hope that it'll trick them into heaviness. At least I had a dream of plums, it means I went to sleep; that's good. But five, six minutes' sleep. That's not good. Who can survive on six minutes of sleep? How can I?

I let the shell drop. Frustration and anger. But there's no use being angry, no use. Think of Venus and the Milky Way and of all the space, all the space in the world, the universe, our bodies, our minds. Everything is made up of space and is more space than it is form. Think about that – you too are more space than you are body. Think about the sky when you look up at night – you see stars, but really what you see is the immense nothingness between stars, and you see how nothingness is the condition for somethingness, how greedy every object is to claim its own arena of space.

Try smiling. Smiling strongly cues to the brain that everything is OK, and brings happiness. Lie here and smile; Venus, the Milky Way, the moon, the bats, the pool, the fathomless repository of a lifetime's memories, the warmth of the bed. Smile. Absurd little row of teeth in the darkness.

Take heart, says something tenacious and laudable – there's still a ten per cent chance you'll sleep, and if you sleep now you can still have five or six hours – plenty. A veritable richness of sleep.

A moment later it revises its estimation down. Six per cent, seven at the most. But that's based on past experience and probability doesn't work like that; every roll of the dice brings equal odds. Throwing four once doesn't lessen the odds of throwing four again, or a hundred times in a row. Every night is a fresh night and a fresh roll of the dice.

In the darkness I fumble again for my conch; it's said that blowing a conch creates a beautiful sound that sees off negative spirits, and I pass my thumb over the blowing end, and bring it to my lips. No sound. Just a salty taste that has no right to be there after so many years of being landlocked at my bedside.

I lie on my front. Maybe I can smuggle sleep in this way, by assuming a position that I never sleep in. Maybe sleep can sneak in before my mind realises what's happening. Maybe I can squash my thrumming heart down to forty beats per minute. I lie in this way for half an hour. Maybe the night won't notice me. Maybe, maybe. Venus, the Milky Way, a plum tree, the mattress, the bats, my bright underwater hands, an aching neck, the lurch of falling asleep, and with the lurch, waking up.

It's well past two. A freight train passes.

The night of my cousin's funeral I'm in a service station café that's soon to close and has a worshipful hush. There's the whirr of a floor cleaner and the metal ting of spatula on catering tray. There's me by the wall of black window and there's me again in the wall of black window; me, and reflection-me.

Reflection-me feeds macaroni cheese into her reflection-mouth, none of which exist – the body, the macaroni cheese, the mouth.

The reflection-body is suspended far away in a thingless black. I ignore it, too hungry. Who knew so firm and buttery a carrot existed on or near a motorway? But then, why has it taken this long? Man has sent a space probe into the rings of Saturn, man has built an underground machine that speeds particles at 299.8 million metres a second to recreate the conditions that existed just after the Big Bang. How could it be only now, in 2018, that a well-cooked carrot has arrived in a service station?

The ghost of me that's floating afield somewhere in the depthless world of reflection is never hungry or full, and has not suffered from weeks without sleep, and doesn't know I've mugged the day to get these thirty minutes for myself between worlds. It doesn't know this dull sense of grief, or this horror when I think: I'm eating macaroni cheese while my cousin, with whom I ran around our grandparents' garden, is buried underground.

Yet I'm warm and calm. I don't want to go home – home is a bed I'm no longer able to sleep in. I don't want to go back – back is my dead cousin. I want to stay; this plastic chair in a vast quiet café by a vast black window feels like the place I've always been looking for.

The day's almost done. There's a pair of men over there finishing up some food, there's a man cleaning the floor, there's a retired-looking couple and a woman at the canteen taking out the scraped trays of shepherd's pie and lasagne. You're all going to die, I think. Compassion surges in me. Can't swallow for the closing up of my throat. You might be taking your fork to a plate of shepherd's pie now, but you, like me, are going to die, and here are the only words I can submit to you:

In the midst of life we are in death.
In the midst of the service station we are in death.
In the midst of the service station we are in life.
In the midst of death we are in the service station.

In the midst of death we are – we are. We *are*.

∞

Some clarifications:

When I don't sleep, which is very often, I don't sleep at all. It's not so much that I'm a bad sleeper these days, it's that I'm a non-sleeper. I am a bad sleeper too, but nights of bad sleep are the good nights, because they involve sleep.

When I don't sleep, it's not that I feel tired so much as assaulted. In the morning after a night of no sleep my eyes are sore and tender and can barely open. My joints ache. There's a taste in my mouth which isn't like any other taste, only like a feeling, and that feeling is defeat. My skull aches evenly across its hemisphere. Pain shoots up to some old scars on the crown of my head. I eye the world with suspicion and everything in it seems to stand back from me with hostility and hatred. There's a force at work that doesn't wish for my wellbeing; it feels personal.

I go up to bed at night, I get beaten up, I come downstairs in the morning. Then I go about the day as if things were normal and I hadn't been beaten up, and everyone else treats me as if I hadn't been beaten up, and that way I survive, but no more than that. If somebody willed your destruction they could do it this way, by taking away your sleep. Of course, it's tried and tested.

I come down late one morning while staying with friends in France. I feel like my face is bruised and that my appearance will appal them, that they'll hide me from their small child. Instead my friend looks at me with infinite compassion and says, *Une petite nuit? Oui*, I say, *une petite nuit, encore*. In this expression, French has it all wrong; nights awake are the longest, largest, most cavernous of things. There is acre upon acre of night, and whole eras come and go, and there isn't another soul to be found on the journey through to morning.

When I don't sleep I spend the night searching the intricacies of my past, trying to find out where I went wrong, trawling through childhood to see if the genesis of the insomnia is there, trying to find the exact thought, thing or happening that turned me from a sleeper to a non-sleeper. I try to find a key to release me from it. I try to solve the logic problem that is now my life. I circle the arena of my mind, its shrinking perimeter, like a polar bear in its grubby blue-white plastic enclosure with fake ice caps and water that turns out to have no depth. I circle and circle. It's 3 a.m., 4 a.m. It's always 3 a.m., 4 a.m. I circle back.

When I don't sleep the world becomes profoundly unsafe. If food were withdrawn, or water, you would feel unsafe; if withdrawn often enough – not long enough to kill you, but often enough to diminish you – you would begin to wonder what the point of life was, if all it does is threaten you with scarcity. There's terror when a basic animal need isn't met. At first you fear death, then a worse thing happens – you fear life. You no longer want your life, not on these terms. When I don't sleep and don't sleep and don't sleep, I don't want my life; neither do I have in me the propulsion (courage? know-how?) to take it. So I have to endure my life when it's unendurable, and this is an impasse.

When I don't sleep I lie still for several hours with my heart pounding, as if evading some beast; when the adrenaline has built in me I break and I get up and hit things, the wall, my head, my head against the wall. I might howl, I might scream. I'll pace, pace, as if trying to stalk down an old, better self that has outrun me.

When I used to sleep I understood nothing about any of this. I knew nothing about what it takes to get through what can't be got through. At night, I'm thrown to the wolves. I only survive by howling like a wolf. This must be true of so many people. Now I know more about that look you see in people's eyes – that homeless man near the bike racks for example, who is slumped every day in faded black clothes on a small luggage trolley, and who in all truth looks like a bin bag, as if he's personified his own absolute sense of redundancy and wastage. If you are being trashed by the machinations of a heedless world, disguise yourself as a bin bag; if you're being savaged by wolves, disguise yourself as a wolf. It's a way of hiding in plain sight.

Sometimes I give him money, which he never asks for, and he watches it fall into the cup by his feet with disinterest. Some days I can't look at him because of that empty gaze when my fifty pence leaves my hand, which seems to say that the days of being helped by money are long gone for him. He's a creature alone; the days of being helped at all are long gone. He's not sitting there because he wants to collect money. He's sitting there because a man's got to be somewhere, because he can't be nowhere. There are days I feel so tired and offended by life that I don't give him money, I don't want to look at him, I wish he'd just disappear, or hurry up and die. The wolf in me wants to attack him for bothering to survive. Why be alive like this? Why can't he just let go, I think. Why can't he just let go?

∞

Maybe it's the menopause, my friend says.

Could it be, already?

Women do stop sleeping well when they hit the menopause.

How do you know if you have?

My friend says to ask my doctor. At the doctor's I sit like a child, with my hands in a loose prayer between my thighs, and my ankles crossed. I always feel like a child the instant I sit before a doctor, and in this case my sense of being one makes it all the more incongruous when I ask about the menopause. I feel flushed and embarrassed to even speak the word, which seems suddenly to designate a club, a band of sisters, a band of mothers, that I'm trying to force my way into.

The doctor says as much. Do you have any other signs of menopause? she asks. Hot flushes, cold night sweats, are your periods still regular?

She says I don't sleep because I'm anxious, and draws attention to my anxiety score derived from a form I filled in.

My body feels suddenly shameful – too old and too young at once, too old to be sitting with this fearful deference to authority and too young to suppose the menopause might be accounting for my troubles. My troubles are just my troubles; I should not try to dignify them with a stage of life, a rite of womanhood. The doctor, herself a woman who must have been through the menopause and presumably carried it off with resilience and not a day's absence from work, is sitting in a posture that mirrors mine – hands between thighs, leaning slightly forward – except in her it's motherly and chastening. It's that forward lean, which says, *now, no more silliness*. It's a primitive tactic for advancing subtly into another's space, just enough that they know who dominates. It feels more combative than it needs to, since my own posture clearly shows I know who dominates. Though of course, that's why it's combative, because my diffidence has provided something to combat. I straighten up and let my hands rest loose on top of my thighs, not between them. They're still linked, though. I would rather unlink them but they won't.

There's not much point in running tests, she says, when I suggest it. They don't show a great deal; hormones are in too much flux and subject to too many variables for a test to be of much use. A test is a snapshot of a biological moment, not an assessment of a state of being.

So there's no way of knowing if my sleep problems could be hormonal, I say, and she says it wouldn't do any good to know in any case since not much can be done, the menopause is something that has to be (she pauses) experienced.

Her choice of word sits oddly between us – not endured or suffered or managed, but experienced, as if it's experience I don't want. It's not suffering I've come here about, it's not that I want to alleviate some suffering but that I want her to make me stop having experiences. In that word is the very sum of her chastening, again, as you would a child: you want the world to be simple, fair and free of all difficulty, but the world isn't that way and the sooner you recognise that I can't immunise you to your own life – the sooner you grow up – the better.

This is surely something women get more than men – this message that they need to learn to put up with things. I read somewhere that women are far more likely to be told by a doctor that their symptoms are stress, while men's symptoms will be investigated and more often referred. By stress, it's meant that women are complicating and compounding their experiences in a way that could be avoidable if only they did breathing and gratitude exercises and stopped being surprised by the inevitabilities of their lives – the feelings of premenstrual rage, the loss of pelvic floor muscles in pregnancy, the loss of bowel control in childbirth, the loss of sleep in menopause, the subjection to various and subtly ubiquitous inequalities and injustices that affect every corner of their lives, the subsuming of oneself in the role of daughterhood to the point that the sense of self becomes so vague as to be virtually derelict and not a self at all, only a roughly amassed set of duties and culpabilities and failures, fought off temporarily by the role of motherhood and all its attendant power, only to return redoubled as the self is once again and spectacularly and irrevocably subsumed by the life of the child, an obliteration not only expected by society, but revered.

The doctor asks me if there's anything else; in doing so she's leaned further forward and is smiling in a way that illustrates how unanimous we are at this point in our conversation, a smile that therefore suggests closure.

If I knew the cause was menopausal I could at least stop looking for other causes, I say. What I mean is I could stop investing my money and time in trying to excavate my being for some emotional artefact that would serve as a clue as to the nature of my self, and in that excavation, painful and invasive as it is, come to a bedrock, the bedrock on which all my fears and neuroses lie, and somehow (in ways I didn't yet understand, but would hopefully come to understand) smash through that bedrock, thereby letting the whole tower of my egoic and troubled self fall through, taking with it my weaknesses, shortcomings, terrors and unhelpful tendencies, among them my insomnia. I don't say any of this to her, only feel there's something in my character that wants in this moment to collapse, something that is asked to exercise the power of an adult and can't. There's only this strange reversion to the powerless panic of childhood – maybe that's one of the artefacts I'm supposed to scrape out from the earth. Maybe that's one of the reasons I don't sleep?

Have you thought about counselling? the doctor asks.

I tell her I've been seeing a counsellor.

And do you think that's a good thing to do?

Good in what way, I want to ask. Good as in wholesome, or as in useful, or as in morally right, the only morally right thing a person can do when they're meanwhile burdening the NHS with their ailments, ailments which originate in the mind? Whichever, I know that the right answer is yes. She wants me to say yes so that I inadvertently admit that my sleeping problems are psychological, not as such biological, and therefore my own responsibility and not hers.

Yes, I say.

Good. So you'll carry on with it?

Why is it – she's thinking – that she has to sit there day after day listening to patients who refuse to take responsibility for their own wellbeing? Why does everyone want a test, a diagnosis, a pill? They want her to wave the magic wand, and it isn't only that she has no wand but that there's no magic in medicine and never was. The days of miraculous cures are gone – she's thinking – or at least her days in believing in them are gone, and now what is she but an agony aunt and a drug dealer. Half of her time is spent not on diagnosing and treating primary illnesses, but on treating all the illnesses caused by side effects of the drugs she's prescribed. She has become a doctor of side effects, treated with more drugs that create more side effects.

Some of it can't be helped – the human body is perishable, medicine imperfect. But then there are all these people who should never have let themselves get to the point of needing medicine, whose problems were preventable and who now want her to take an action that will compensate for the actions they didn't take themselves. People in Syria can sleep with bombs falling, why can't you sleep on your king-size mattress with your winter-togged duvet and your kelp-scented hair on a fake-down pillow under a bomb-free sky? What pea disrupts your sleep, princess? A passing Audi? What paucity and fragility of spirit has left you relying on drugs to do that which is the natural inheritance of all animals everywhere and forever? But prescribe drugs she must, because that's what they want. People are rattling with drugs, you can hear it when they walk in. Maybe they don't even want to get better, they've got used to the sad prestige of being unwell. They want her to both acknowledge how magnificently, uniquely unwell they are and to reassure them that despite this they won't have undue pain and won't die.

I've told her yes, I'll carry on with the counselling, and will meditate every day and try more relaxation techniques at bedtime, and while I'm speaking she's gazing at the computer screen, then turns back to me and cocks her head.

No catastrophising, she says softly.

No catastrophising, I say.

I'm not sure now if I feel like a child or a person standing in front of a magistrate in a district court, someone promising to change her ways and be a good citizen and stop being a burden on society. The child is meek and innocent, the person in court meek and guilty. I can't decide which I am.

The doctor seems pleased in a muted way. I want to tell her that the counselling, meditation and relaxation techniques that I already do, every day, aren't improving my sleep and are increasing my sense of failure, since now I not only fail at sleeping but also at meditating, relaxing and being counselled. I look out of the tall sash window and across the gardens, river, railway line and canal to the hills beyond, and see the huge Georgian building that I used to live in, on that hill. Thinking about myself there is like reading a lifestyle magazine article about another person, someone you're supposed to admire.

I do admire her, but more for being young than for any particular achievement, and it strikes me that nothing I've ever done was an achievement as such, it was just an outcome of a set of conditions that made me who I was but weren't of my doing. Being young, sleeping well, charged with ambitious energy – none of that was of my doing, just as being middle-aged and sleeping badly and finding the act of novel writing pointless is none of my doing. It feels a relief to realise this. I want to ask the doctor how she feels about being a woman of her age, about the loss of beauty and of the power of beauty – though you can't ask somebody a question like that for fear of offence. You would have to qualify that by beauty you mean obvious, youthful beauty, and that there are other types; you'd then have to explain that you do think they have that other type. In the doctor's case, she does. Her back is exceptionally upright, her head carried with elegance, her hair pulled back in the same kind of ponytail she might have had when she was ten; she has a sleepiness about her but also the carriage of her back makes her seem very alert, and it's the incongruity of those two things that make her striking.

If you want I can offer you a blood test, she says, and it's an assertion and concession of power at once – to offer the very thing someone asked for and which you'd previously withheld, and to offer it because it's a gift you've finally decided to give, a pointless gift you will give, not because you must, but because you can.

I say yes, please, I do want. By now – and somehow as a result of looking out of the window and considering my old self in that grand rented flat – I've come to a place of almost certain recognition that there's no dawning of menopause in me, not yet, or that if there is it isn't the cause of my sleeplessness. I've never felt it was, I only came to the doctor about it because my friend said so – and not just my friend, several people, so that it felt negligent and churlish of me not to at least ask. Now I've asked, and the asking of the question has also been the negation of it. It's as if I've had to beg to be considered for membership of a club I don't want to join, and in the begging I've seen that all I want is reassurance that there's no need to beg.

I dread the idea of being menopausal. I dread the passage into this last phase of life. There's a vivid image of myself as a twelve year old getting my first period in the childhood home of Shakespeare's wife, Anne Hathaway, in Stratford, while a guide explained the origin of the phrase 'turning the tables'. Menopause feels like a betrayal of that girl, though I'm not sure why. Maybe because I haven't had children, and so the process that began that day has never fulfilled itself, and maybe for that reason I'll never meet my menopause and old age with a great level of acceptance; there will always be a feeling of unfinished business.

Still, I say yes to the blood test, since it's what I came here asking for. This mysterious and autonomous shifting of hormones is a kind of inner ghost-life that's been at work in me all my life, and I have a longing now to get a glimpse of it. I look out of that tall window again. All I ever seem to feel these days is the disappearance of who I think I am. I would like to see myself, even if it's only a snapshot that diagnoses nothing; I don't, in fact, care at all for a diagnosis any more. And when, a fortnight later, I see the tube full of my burgundy blood, there's an unexpected surge of some feeling I can't identify. I'm moved by it. It feels idiotic to be moved by a tube of your own blood, yet I am – moved by and possessive of it.

Then a week later when the test results come back normal it points towards what I already know, which is that my sleeplessness is psychological. I must carry on being the archaeologist of myself, digging around, seeing if I can excavate the problem and with it the solution – when in truth I am afraid of myself, not of what I might uncover, but of managing to uncover nothing.

∞

There was once a girl.

There was once a girl aged something like twelve.

Had a dog.

Had a dog.

A dog of big, bewitching gentleness. Of long black and brown coat and swift speed and big carnivorous teeth and nothing-ever-but-gentleness. A dog caught up in the chaotic tit for tat of divorce.

It was half term. The girl was visiting her dad, who'd been left with the custody of the dog, or should I say demanded the custody of the dog given that it was the mum's dog, and he either wanted to keep this living part of her or wanted to punish this living part of her; I don't know. It was half term and the girl and her sister were staying with the dad for the week.

The dog didn't live with the dad, despite his demand for custody, because the dad lived with the new wife, just around the corner, and the new wife didn't like anything that had anything to do with the old wife. The dog lived in the house that had once, only two or so years before, been a warm, busy home to a family of four: dad, mum, daughter, daughter. Now the house was empty; nobody lived there but the dog and its astonishingly multiplying fleas.

The dad came each day to feed it, and most days to walk it, but there were at least twenty-three hours in every day that the dog now spent alone. The neighbours complained that it howled most of the day and all of the night – their complaint wasn't only because of the disturbance to them, but because they were alarmed that a creature should be abandoned in this way. The dad said he'd try to visit the dog more often, but it was difficult, what with a business to run and new wife and new stepchildren and new stepdogs, plus the occasional visitations of old actual children.

In the school holidays the girl and her sister made the three-hour journey from their mum's house to visit the dad. This half-term holiday, as with every holiday, when the girl visited, she spent all her time at the old house with the dog. She didn't feel welcome at the new wife's house, and didn't like it anyhow – it smelt of poverty and of urine and of lingering cooked dinners. She walked the dog, she sat for hours stroking the silken patch between the dog's ears, or the pink, hairless patch on the belly, which the dog loved. She talked at length to the dog about how things were. She tried crushing the fleas between her fingers; she found the best way to kill them was to fill the bathroom sink with water and drown them. She lay down with the dog on the flea-flocked carpet and they slept. When it came to the end of the day and she had to go, she would be bitten from head to foot. It was of no consequence.

A year of this. This half term, however, was the last of it. The girl had appealed so strongly to her mum, and her mum to her dad, that it was agreed, after a miserable year of this arrangement, that the dog would come to live with the girl, the girl's sister, and the mum. When the girl and her sister went home on the Sunday, the dog would go with them and they'd all live together, in the mum's new house.

This half term the girl had done as always; spent all day every day with the dog, and had told the dog the plan. Told it many times, clearly, plainly, so that the dog would understand that it wasn't some fancy, some childish wish, but a reality agreed upon. Just as well, because by Wednesday the dog was ill. The girl could see this. It wouldn't eat, and where it would usually have defied its Alsatian largeness with a balletic, bounding greeting when the girl walked through the door, a bounding of pure joy, it now lifted only its head. Some kind of brokenness of spirit, the girl thought, which would have been tragic if not for the soonness of relief. She told the dog not to worry. She left at the end of that day with reassurances. Not to worry. Not to worry.

The next day the dog still wouldn't eat, nor drink. It was listless. Its nose was warm and dry; this was all the girl knew about dog health – if the nose was cool and wet the dog was well, and if the nose was warm and dry it wasn't. She knew, regardless of the nose, that the dog wasn't well, but the nose seemed to confirm it as outward proof. She went to the next-door neighbour, since the dad was at work and she didn't know how to contact him. The neighbour came to look, and called the vet. The vet came. He glanced around the abandoned living room with its fleas, its dust, its cold stale smell, then knelt and administered to the dog with a terrible tenderness that made the girl want to cry. He decided the dog had a kidney infection and should be encouraged to drink as often as possible. He gave the girl some pills to give the dog. Before he left he told the girl, and the neighbour, that the dog should not, under any circumstances, be left alone.

That night, for the first time, the girl stayed in the house with the dog. Even though it had been her home since birth and the house of all her firsts – first word, first tooth, first day at school, first sighting of imaginary friend, first book independently read – she didn't like to stay in it any more. With all its furniture in place, its bedrooms laid out for a family of four, its beds still made, the lace tablecloth on the table that belonged to her great-granddad, the mum's candelabra on top of that, inappropriately grand for the three-bed semi, the horse and cart on the windowsill, the statue of John Wayne on the shelf, the mum's drawings on the kitchen wall, the dad's cartoons next to them. Everything was as it had been except untouched. Everything had a film of grime. She was somehow afraid of the house, of going upstairs in the dark. She slept downstairs on the sofa, next to the dog, with her hand on the dog's back.

There was no choice, the next day, but for the dad to do what did not come naturally to him, and stand up to his new wife. He insisted that the dog should be allowed into the new wife's house. The dog was barely moving by now, and when the girl stroked the patch between its ears there was only a twitch of its ears or brows, which seemed to the girl to be small gestures of gratitude, but no longer pleasure. She told it that there were only two more days; the day after tomorrow the dog wouldn't have to bear this house, it would be going home with her. Just two more days.

By this time, the girl knew that the dog was dying. If she'd been honest with herself, she'd known it from the very first moment she walked in the house two days before, when the dog didn't bound. When she saw the dog rise slowly, tail wagging, there'd been a heaviness in her own legs, not a weakness, just a slight heaviness, that was the heaviness of predictability. The knowledge of events to come. It had always been her legs that suffered; there had been strange growing pains for years that had made her temporarily unable to walk, as if anticipating old age, or future grief. She wondered if her legs had known all along, from birth, that her mum would leave, that her dog would be tortured this way and die. Could legs know such things? Well, maybe.

She didn't want the dog to go to the new wife's house. She couldn't picture it there, with the other scrawny dogs that she and her sister called, unimaginatively, the rats, she couldn't picture its magnificence in that stale, brown room. But she also did want the dog to go there; she wanted everyone to see that the dog was ill and to understand, when it died, that they'd killed it. The dog crawled behind the new wife's sofa and lay still. It wouldn't drink. The vet was called again, and this time when he left, the house was very quiet and even the new wife, who only ever bore the expression of a viper, looked softer and pale.

On Halloween morning, the Saturday, the dog died. That night the dad's brother – the girl's uncle – was having a Halloween party. The new wife didn't want the dad to go, and the dad, who had wanted to go, had already promised her, sulkily, that he wouldn't. The girl remembered days when the dad had seemed strong, a giant to her, a man who could leapfrog over a five-foot post.

The dog's death took all the air out of the world. Its body was driven to the vet's and left there; it had probably been in pain for some time, a week or two or three, the vet said. But dogs are resilient; they want to please their owners. The dad cried; the girl had never seen her dad cry before and she both wished that he would stop and wished that he would never stop. Her sister had never been attached to the dog, but she cried briefly before trying, with an expression of faraway torment, to be a comfort, as was her way.

In the last two years or so, the girl had learned a lot about the way adults treat each other, the blame they have for one another, the blame she felt towards herself for their and her own unhappiness; it had seemed to her that if some of it was her fault then some of it could be fixed by her. That Halloween, she saw the dad blame his new wife for the dog's death, and saw the new wife blame the dad for caring more about the dog's death than he did about her. The girl wanted only to be on her own in the old house, the dog's house as she now saw it, to touch the things the dog had touched, to collect some of its hair from the carpet and take it with her, to sit among its fleas.

That evening the dad, the girl and her sister went to the Halloween party. Everybody at the party agreed that the dad needed to be there, and each time the new wife phoned, a different person answered to tell her that the dad needed to be there, at his own brother's party, to be with his family on such a sad day, when he'd had such a tough time of it these last two years, when his wife had left him and the children, left him to cope with two young girls, then eventually the girls had gone too, re-appearing in the school holidays for too short a time. Off his girls were going the next day back to their mum's, poor man having such a rough day, he needed to have some time to spend with them.

When the dad, the girl and her sister walked back to the new wife's house that night after the party, with the girl on one side of the staggering dad and the sister on the other, they came to the gate that opened into a small, grassless front garden, and found all of the dad's things in front of the door and window, from where they had been hurled.

They walked, the dad now suddenly less staggering, to the old house, went in. The girl didn't go to the kitchen, where the dog's untouched water bowl was, and the old towel the dog had used for a bed. It was cold in the house. They went up to the rooms they'd always gone to before – the girl remembering how she'd used to imagine her bed was a rowing boat on a vast night-time sea – and just as they'd used to do in these rooms for all those years, they slept.

∞

Months ago I had a dream that I was in a high-speed shuttle in a hot narrow tube for an untold time, my satchel pressed to my chest while a voice barked an order not to speak, to ask no questions, to expect nothing. I was sardined with a hundred unknown others whose fear formed a film of sweat on the ceiling of our tube, and there was a certain wobble to our hurtle, a sense that the space we flew through wasn't the effortless path to a better place but a thrust into grit, beyond which – what? Who could say?

I woke up and thought, Thank god that was a dream. A moment later, What if that was a glimpse of death?

I couldn't shake the feeling off. Months later, I still can't shake the feeling off.

I call my mother and say, Comfort me, protect me from this outcome. She says, Death is beautiful, I know it, don't worry. I say, How do you know, you don't know. She says, I just know.

∞

3 a.m.:

The long trail of the freight train snags the night. Something has been torn (how apt, that phrase, 'morning has broken') – it won't be mended now until night falls again. From here there will be more freight trains, then the first flight passing overhead at around four, and at five or five thirty the traffic will start up, and from there our hyperactive little planet will flare once more to life. At three, the first ember has already taken. In reality, for those awake enough to register it, there is about an hour of night at most – somewhere between two and three, a brief lull between one day dwindling and the next awakening.

I get up. Current wisdom is conflicted on this. Some sleep regimes say you should get up if you're still awake after twenty minutes, so that you don't associate bed with sleeplessness. Others say you should stay in bed regardless, so that you don't signal to the body that it's normal to be up in the night; instead you stay in bed and accept what comes.

Inherently inert at night, and clinging on to some idea of myself as a good sleeper, I'm much more predisposed to the latter. Tonight, though, I get up. I'm restless. I make a cup of tea. Absolutely no sleep regimes advocate having a caffeinated drink at 3 a.m. but I did it once and went straight to sleep afterwards, so occasionally I try it just in case it works again, which it never has.

There's a line from a Philip Larkin poem that comes to me. I don't know the poem first-hand, I found it in a book about poetry I've recently read – something about a million-petalled flower. Sitting on the sofa in my underwear, drinking tea, I do the other thing no sleep regime advocates – I go online. There is the poem, in which Larkin remarks on the oblivion of death. It is 'only oblivion', he says:

We had it before, but then it was going to end,
And was all the time merging with a unique
   endeavour
To bring to bloom the million-petalled flower
Of being here.

It feels like a bell ringing distantly, like the heralding of company in what you thought was a desert or an abyss. Suddenly I don't feel lonely, I feel elated, and everything is soft and full of echoes and resonance. Then I think of a line from another poem by Jack Underwood, that describes the elation of holding a newborn baby: 'I can feel my socks being on' he writes. And when I read it I can feel my socks being on, even if I'm not wearing any. Poetry can turn phrases that rotate the world, too small a rotation to cause a public commotion but enough to knock a solitary life a fraction off its axis, such that it will never quite be the same again. It's that turn of phrase – 'the million-petalled flower of being here' – that knocks my axis now. After years of labouring over Buddhist, Hindu, Christian teachings that try to get me to some finishing line of selfhood, this phrase of Larkin's is a steroid straight to the veins. I've sprinted past my old labouring self and have arrived at the finishing line, which of course doesn't exist, which turns out to be an ever-replenishing starting point. My life, all life, opens out in accelerated footage of growth. It doesn't feel like it could ever stop, and that's the trick of life – it seems so abundant, and even while we're watching it die all around us it's whispering in our ears sweet-nothings of plenitude.

At around half past three I go back to bed. To have come this far through the night and feel in some way peaceful is surely an augur for sleep. Also, I'm cold. Getting into bed, nestling down, there are a few minutes of contentment that remind me of how it always used to be. I used to love going to bed. Remember that now. My life, so convoluted and iterative and searching, is nothing more complex or more simple than the million-petalled flower of being here. I am alive, I think, as if I've just discovered an extraordinary fact. I can feel my life being on.

∞

Here: my mother. Singing along to 'The Windmills of Your Mind' as she does the housework. Polishing her silver candelabra and the matching silver goblets. Me, small, listening.

Round, like a circle in a spiral, like a wheel within a wheel, never ending or beginning in an ever-spinning reel.

Something in my brain responding to the words whose collective meaning I couldn't comprehend, but following the repetitions and the melody as if along a path corkscrewing around a mountain. The living room would turn strange. I'd load up the wooden cart with marbles, adjust the bridle of the china Shire horse – this was the ornamental horse and cart everyone had in the 80s – and tsk tsk the horse on. Off to market! My mum's singing in the background would give rise to random images. Water swirling down a drain. Bedtimes. The willow tree. The woods we walked in. *Like a tunnel that you follow to a tunnel of its own.* The melody of that song going nowhere, a pendulum rocking back and forth, back and forth. The china horse trundling across our light green carpet.

∞

Think of a sentence:

> One day I'd like to write a story about a man who, while robbing a cash machine, loses his wedding ring and has to go back for it because his wife, a terrifying individual whose material needs have driven him to crime, will no doubt kill him if the ring is lost.

A sentence with multiple clauses, one clause buried within another like Russian dolls. If we take each doll out and line them up we get:

> One day I'd like to write a story.
> The story is about a man.
> A man robs a cash machine.
> A man loses his wedding ring.
> A man goes back to the cash machine for his wedding ring.
> A man has a wife.
> The wife is terrifying.
> The wife has many material needs.
> The man is driven to crime by his wife.
> The ring must not get lost.
> The wife could kill the man.

We tend to speak in sentences of multiple clauses, not in clauses that have been separated out. Noam Chomsky has called these multiple clauses instances of recursion, and he thinks they're what define human language. They reflect our unique ability to position a thought inside a thought, to move from the immediate to the abstract, to infinite other places and times. A circle in a spiral, a wheel within a wheel; a tunnel that you follow to a tunnel of its own. In theory, an infinitely long, recursive sentence is possible, says Chomsky; there is no limit to the mind's capacity to embed one thought inside another. Our language is recursive because our minds are recursive. Infinitely windmilling.

But then came studies on the Pirahã people of the Brazilian Amazon, who do not make recursive sentences. Their language doesn't permit them to make the sentence I made above, or even something like *When it rains I'll take shelter*. For the Pirahã it would have to be *It rains. I take shelter*. They don't embed a thought inside a thought, nor travel from one time or place to another within a single sentence.

When it rains, unless I take shelter, I get wet.

Unless I want to get wet, I take shelter when it rains.

So that I stay dry when it rains, I take shelter.

For the Pirahã tribe there are no sentences like these – there is none of this restless ranging from one hypothesis to another. Instead, *It rains. I take shelter*. Or, *I take shelter. I don't get wet*. Or, *I take shelter. I stay dry*.

The Pirahã seem incapable of abstraction. They seem literal in the extreme – their ability to learn new grammar rules through a computerised game, by predicting which way an icon of a monkey would go when a type of sentence was generated, was thwarted in almost every case by their inability to see the monkey as real, and therefore to care what it would do next. They became fascinated and distracted by the icon, or by the colours on the screen. One of them fell asleep in the middle of the test. 'They don't do new things' was the repeated assertion of Daniel Everett, the only westerner who has ever got anywhere near knowing and understanding the Pirahã language and culture. They don't tell stories. They don't make art. They have no supernatural or transcendental beliefs. They don't have individual or collective memories that go back more than one or two generations. They don't have fixed words for colours. They don't have numbers.

Yet they are a bright, alert, capable, witty people who are one of the only tribes in the world to have survived – largely in the jungle – without any concession to the modern world. A meal might involve sucking the brains from a just-killed rat. A house is fronds of palm or a piece of leather strung over four sticks in the ground. They have no possessions. Their language might involve speaking, but it might also occur through whistling, singing or humming. And their experience of the present moment is seemingly absolute. 'The Pirahã's excitement at seeing a canoe go around a river bend is hard to describe,' Everett writes. 'They see this almost as travelling into another dimension.'[6]

There is a Pirahã word that Everett heard often and couldn't deduce the meaning of: *xibipiio*. Sometimes it would be a noun, sometimes a verb, sometimes an adjective or adverb. So and so would xibipiio go upriver, and xibipiio come back. The fire flame would be xibipiio-ing. Over time Everett realised that it designated a concept, something like *going in and out of experience* – 'crossing the border between experience and non-experience'. Anything not in the here and now disappears from experience, it xibipiios, and arrives back in experience as once again the here and now. There isn't a 'there' or a 'then', there are just the things xibipiio-ing in and out of the here and now.

There is no past or future tense as such in Pirahã; the language has two tense-like morphemes – remote things (not here and now) are appended by -*a* and proximate things (here and now) by -*i*. These morphemes

---

[6] This and every of Everett's quotations here is from his paper 'Cultural Constraints on Grammar and Cognition in Pirahã'. If you find the Pirahã interesting, this, and his other writings, are very worth reading and so much better at illuminating the tribe's culture and language than my attempts could ever be.

don't so much describe time as whether the thing spoken about is in the speaker's direct experience or not. The Pirahã language doesn't lay experiences out on a past–present–future continuum as almost every other language does. In English we can place events quite precisely on this continuum: it had rained, it rained, it has rained, it rains, it is raining, it will rain, it will have rained. The Pirahã can only say whether the rain is proximate (here) or not.

They can then modify a verb to qualify the claims they make about it. If they say 'It rained in the night', the verb 'rain' will be modified by one of three morphemes to convey how they know it rained, i.e. whether they heard about it (someone told them), deduced it (saw the ground was wet in the morning), or saw/heard it for themselves. The Pirahã language and culture is not only literal but evidence-based. How do you know something happened? If the line of hearsay becomes too long, involving too many steps away from experience, the thing is no longer deemed to be of any importance to speak or think about. This is why they don't have transcendental beliefs or collective memories and stories and myths that go back generations.

What a thing this is, to be so firmly entrenched in the here and now. What a thing. We are, I am, spread chaotically in time. Flung about. I can leap thirty-seven years in a moment; I can be six again, listening to my mum singing while she cleans the silver candelabra she treasures, that reminds her of a life she doesn't have. I can sidestep into another possible version of myself now, one who made different, better decisions. I can rest my entire life on the cranky hinge of the word 'if'. My life is when and until and yesterday and tomorrow and a minute ago and next year and then and again and forever and never.

Time leaks everywhere into English, some ten per cent of the most commonly used words are expressions of time. The Pirahã language has almost no words that depict time. This is all of them: another day; now; already; day; night; low water; high water; full moon; during the day; noon; sunset/sunrise; early morning, before sunrise. Their words for these are literally descriptive – the expression for day is 'in sun', for noon 'in sun big be' and for night 'be at fire'.

Are there whole slices and movements of time that the Pirahã people don't experience, then? If they can only speak in terms of 'another day', do they not experience 'yesterday' and 'a year ago' as different things? If something doesn't exist in a language, does it also not exist in the minds of those who speak the language?

I wondered that when I tried to teach the perfect tense to Japanese students; there isn't a perfect tense in Japanese. When I taught the sentence *I have eaten* I got blank looks, incomprehension. Why not just say *I ate*? Why say *I have been to Europe* when you could just say *I went to Europe*? I tried to illustrate: *I ate* (before, at some time you need to specify – this morning, all day yesterday); *I have eaten* (just now, I'm still full). Blank looks, incomprehension. In the perfect tense a period of time opens out, the past, not as separate from the present, but running up to and meeting the present. I have eaten; we've danced all night; it's been a year. Do the Japanese not experience that segment of time? Or is it that they deal with it in other linguistic ways, or by inference and context?

Everett described the Pirahã's mode of being as 'live here and now'. If you live here and now, you don't need recursion in language because there's no conceptual need to join together ideas or states according to their order in time, or in terms of which causes which, or in terms of hypothetical outcomes. You don't need a past or future tense if you're living only now. You don't need a large stock of words that try to nail down instances of time along a horizontal continuum from the distant past to the distant future, a continuum that also has an enormous elastic stretch into the vertical planes of virtual time, time as it intersects with space, time as happening elsewhere, real or imagined.

What would it be like to be a person of the Pirahã tribe? How would it be to not experience that continuum? For one's mind to not be an infinitely recursive wheel within a wheel? It feels in some ways a relief, even to imagine such a mode of living, but it feels almost non-human too. And yet there the Pirahã are, as human as human can be. I can't imagine it. I can't imagine being anything but submersed in time, it ticking in every cell.

Time has always felt to me so alive and strange; even when I was a child listening to my mother singing 'The Windmills of Your Mind' I knew something odd was going on. My hands, transferring marbles in and out of the cart, would feel warm and have the sensation of swelling to ten times their size. I knew that the song was addressing something ungraspable but intimate. Our minds are lost in space and time. Or not lost, I don't know, maybe when you've gone down enough wormholes and black holes and opened into enough new realities there's no longer a question of being lost. It's only when you get stuck in the black holes and wormholes that you begin to feel lost.

Sometimes time, for me, is a medium with a sort of viscosity, like water, or like oil, or like mud, depending on how it impacts on me. I move through it with differing degrees of ease and difficulty, and am aware of it getting lumpier, less consistent, as I get older. I see it reorganising my face and body, shapes shifting – a youthful soft line becomes harsh and old, a youthful harsh line soft and old. I see it dismantle people I love. Sometimes it's like a surface I hit when I desperately want something to happen and am tired of waiting. Then I watch the clock and the second hand appears to quiver long and lingering between every shift. Other times it moves around the clock face, fleet and even, as if helped by a tail wind.

It's an abundance, so much of it; a king-size duvet on a single bed that I can grasp in fistfuls. Then it's like scratching at barren ground; not enough of it to make anything, do anything. It's darkness. My life appears as shapes within it, ones that come and go. It's a horse I must lasso. I'm the horse and it has me lassoed.

St Augustine asked: what is time but a set of nothings? The 'no longer' and the 'not yet' separated by the vanishing now. Is that where the Pirahã live, in a vanishing now? Nights are spent thinking about this. I try to imagine a life without narrative, which is easier in the night, because the night is itself without narrative – the way the hours move, less like a stream flowing some-where and more like water swilling in a shallow pool, until suddenly the pool is drained and it's morning. Do they, the Pirahã? Live in a vanishing now?

I don't know if St Augustine is right except on the level of technicality; the past itself might be no-longer, and the future itself not-yet, but my thoughts and feel-ings about the past are here, now, as I lie awake remem-bering my childhood bed as a rowing boat, or remem-bering my mother singing, and my thoughts and feelings about the future are here, now, as I envisage years of this, being awake all night, worrying and won-dering and envisaging years more. That past isn't no-longer if it's alive in me now, and by the same token that future isn't not-yet. Both are now; in imagination, yes, but through imagination they arrive as physical fact, in my neural pathways, and in my emotions whose flavour and intensity affect the rapidity of my heartbeat and the rhythm of my breathing. Lying here awake, confronting a future that will bring years more of lying here awake, I've made a fist to protect myself; there are little moons incised on my palms where my nails have dug in. These little moons aren't not-yet, they're here, my fear of the future really put them here. The future is now.

As for the continual vanishing of the now, well, here is also the continual birth of the now. A live birth, from a living now; there are no deaths, there's no hiatus. It seems to me that now is the largest, most predictable and most durable of all things, and that the question isn't so much: what is time but a set of nothings? But more: what is time but an indomitable something? An unscalable wall of now. When I think of the Pirahã I don't imagine them cresting the brink of a collapsing moment, each step bringing an existential vertigo. I imagine them fishing, skinning animals, drinking, painting their faces, building shelter. *It rains. We stay dry.* Their here and now seems as solid to me as one brick – *it rains* – laid on another – *we stay dry.*

What *would* it be like to live and think like the Pirahã? For the world to be continually xibipiio-ing? No mad spooling out of events through time, all chain-linked and dragged each by the next, one event causing another, one event blamed for another, one past pain locked into a present pain to cause future pain; no. No things crossing the boundary from experience to non-experience. Just things disappearing and reappearing around the bend of the river.

I was ill once and in pain – long ago, in my early twenties. It was a kidney infection; in moments of almost hallucinatory pain it occurred to me I was being granted a way of knowing in some sense what my dog knew back when she'd suffered the same, or it was a way of making recompense for her suffering. It felt that my kidneys were the size of rugby balls, the pain distorting and hijacking my perception. It was a hot, solid, ceaseless ache that left me hardly able to move. Then, one night, lying in my makeshift bed on the living-room floor, I thought I'd died. All the pain had suddenly gone and my body was dense but light, like an air-filled lung, and when I moved my arm to look at my hand I saw it with complete equanimity. Am I dead, I asked, am I dead? I couldn't know. I was only curious, not at all afraid.

I watched the clock on the video and it was moving, and I wondered what that meant. It could be moving in an afterlife. Its numbers were just numbers. They bore no relationship to me. They weren't tugging in a forwards direction, they were just things gently changing, rearranging, in the same way that the clouds rearrange, and they were rearranging in a vast stillness. They were xibipiio-ing. Only: here I am. Then: here I am. Then: here I am.

Is that akin to the Pirahã's experience of time? Is that where the dance is, the dance T. S. Eliot told us about when we read *Four Quartets* as uncomprehending teenagers? *At the still point, there the dance is.* My painless night watching the video clock was the most serene I've ever known, and yet there the dance was – an extreme aliveness even as I thought I was dead. The aliveness I felt was, I think, some reverb happening in sudden stillness. And in fact the feeling that I might be dead came from the new awareness of being alive – not the usual awareness of doing this or that, or of the pain in my kidney, or being sleepy or hot, but an awareness that there was a thing beyond all this that was alive, and that thing was me. Now that there wasn't any pain or sleepiness or heat to mask it, I could know it directly, and now that I knew it I also knew the possibility of not-it. Life and death were one sphere with a continuous surface.

I watched the video clock that night for hours, and it was only by seeing that the minutes were following evenly on from each other in a plausible, predictable and sustained way that I came, eventually, to doubt being dead. I watched the two-fold working of time on the digital display – the undulation of the minutes as they built up and were knocked back to zero, and the steady accumulation of hours stacked one on top of the other, and under this persistent, silent double advance my stillness was eroded, a fortress that had given way to siege.

In those erosions, pain came slowly in, then thirst, and tiredness. I felt the weight of time again, its perpetual nagging. Time kicks, kicks, kicks its way in with the tip of a toe. Time is the thing that breaks apart life from death, eases apart their embrace. Time, not life, is what we live. Time, not life, is what runs out. Time pushes death over there, where we can see it, and then offers itself as finite protection. Time is the breeding ground of fear and despair.

Do the Pirahã fail to sleep? Do they worry? Do they ever pace the floor? It was night, I think now, filled with hopeless rage. It was Tuesday night and now it's Wednesday morning. Tuesday has become Wednesday and not a shred of sleep has separated out the two. How can I survive these forty-hour days? All these minutes of the night and day, time is living me into submission; I give up, I say into the darkness and then into the morning light, I give up.

I have been awake all night and now it's morning, say I. Panic building, a story of woe unfurling. *I have been awake all night, all the long night, and now it's morning. It was Tuesday and I didn't sleep and now it's Wednesday.*

It is night. I don't sleep. It is morning, say the Pirahã, for whom this, with these recursions, is impossible. For whom the past has just flickered out of experience, gone.

It is Tuesday, they might say, with factual unrecursive ease, with no wind of time to turn the windmills of their minds. *It is Tuesday. I don't sleep. It is Wednesday.*

∞

We'll go to Wales.

We won't take much, just the whole car full. It's January. We'll walk by the sea. We'll swim in the sea? Wetsuits in, playing cards, Scrabble just in case, laptops, books, wellies, Netflix log-in, washing powder, fire lighters, logs, camera, bikes. Not bikes. Bikes. Bikes in. Anyone can sleep in Wales. It's dark and cold and there's nothing to do. We'll sleep in Wales, sleep for England.

We'll hear the stream. We'll look out in the morning where we parked wonkily in the dark and we still won't see the stream but we'll hear it, and we'll see the rain. We'll light the fire. Matches. Matches. Matches? We'll walk to the shop to buy matches. We'll light the fire and watch the flames, we'll feel like Tarzan and Jane. Me Tarzan, you Jane.

We'll cook our repertoire: Monday pasta, Tuesday chilli, Wednesday baked potatoes, Thursday pasta again, Friday curry. We won't make curry, there aren't any spices, we'll make it into a pasta sauce instead. Pasta again. Saturday out. Sunday baked potatoes again. Monday repeat. There's paprika. We'll add that to everything. We'll juice carrots: eight carrots, two centimetres of juice. We'll juice red cabbage. We won't juice red cabbage again.

We'll walk on the cliffs. We'll wrap our heads in scarves against the wind. We'll walk for hours above the roaring sea. We'll see a seal, no, an otter. An otter? An otter! We'll watch a swimmer in the bay and pretend to be sad about not having our wetsuits. We'll think of them hanging up at the house like new year's resolutions. We'll see herons and we'll disappoint a swan with our breadlessness. We'll regret not bringing food, for ourselves as much as for the swan. We never bring food, why do we never bring food? One day, we'll buy a proper flask that keeps things hot. We'll buy Nordic walking poles and gaiters and a Labrador. We'll live by the sea, one of these days.

We'll watch the rain. We'll hear the rain. We'll see the rain, we'll see the rain make lakes of fields. We'll get wet and covered in cow shit. We'll see the stream gush above the bridge. We'll drive two hours to see a house we'll never buy, and have to turn back half a mile before it because the road is flooded. We won't buy that, we'll say. It floods.

Just before dusk we'll drive up into a nature reserve that boasts good murmurations. We'll wait for two hours in the merciless grey of midwinter and see a blue tit and two woodpeckers. Then it'll get dark and we'll go home. Not home, but home so to speak.

We'll work; we'll vanish each into our screen-worlds, we'll surface to put a log on the fire, we'll turn the heating up, we'll feel bad and turn it down, we'll listen to the logs hiss damply, we'll turn the heating back up. Off to the shop: some bad bread and more matches. A *Guardian* to get the flames going. We'll investigate the upturned boat in the garden, an altar to someone's little gods. Shells, stones, plastic figures, a length of rope, incense holders. We'll argue over a bird. Bullfinch. No way, chaffinch. Bullfinch. Not pink enough. Female one. Chaffinch. Bullfinch. Chaffinch. You're deluded. Whatever. We'll play blackjack without speaking. You'll win, you'll win, you'll win, I'll win, you'll win.

We'll go to bed, we'll choose which room. This night this one, that night that. We'll lie in perfect darkness. The darkness is perfect, we'll say. Yes, perfect. We won't give a thought to the number 3 bus that's going at this moment past our bedroom at home. We won't give a thought to the planes, the trains, the hum of our neighbour's boiler.

We'll wonder why the hurtling of the wind and the hammering of the rain feel like silence. Sometimes – bad nights – we'll be up, 3 a.m., 4 a.m., battling off the demons. My fucking father, I'll say, in the grip of a sudden unbidden memory. He killed my dog. He drove my mother away and he killed my dog. Then we'll watch while the blackness and silence swallow the rage. Forgiveness will come, it always does – of my dad, of the past, because it's easier to live reconciled to your life than to be counting the losses. We'll look out of the window at the beautiful never-ending rain, the smell of sanded wood, the generous dark of dawn, the struggle of the stream. We'll wonder why it feels more like home than home. Why lying awake here brings memories of being a child. Why lying awake has its own grace. Why sleep is deeper and dreamless when it comes.

We'll pack up the car. We'll shove everything around the untouched bikes. Next time, we'll say, about the wetsuits. We'll leave first thing, before it's light, before the robins and bullfinches and whatevers are up. We'll drive the long way, to see the sea one more time; we'll wonder what it is about the sea. Then we'll press home, fast as we can to beat the traffic, we'll put music on and sing quietly along. The only music in the car is from the 90s, from the age of CDs, dated music which we'll pretend to listen to ironically. We'll each kid ourselves, privately, that we're back there in the past, in all our various near-far pasts. We'll watch the wipers chop-chop-chopping back the rain. Endless rain, we'll sing, endless rain.

———

Proliferations of love. Vows and confidences and wedding bands, long nights up with the children, years of devotion, doing your best. Now, suddenly he's thinking. He's thinking of hills for some reason, not mountains but soft hills and thunderstorms and David Bowie on stage in Berlin with his hair fluttering and *The Women of Renaissance Ferrara* and a drum beat and twenties spewing from a cash machine and his mother by the sea and James's undeniable smile and there's James in front of him now and looking at him feels like something rushing through him, a wind blowing open a multitude of doors. That's what it feels like. That all his doors have blown open.

/

It's just gone ten on a Tuesday in early July, the bright light of day. He waits for the green man before crossing the road. He'd normally weave across, hands in pockets looking straight ahead, but there's something in this moment about being a risk-averse, law-abiding citizen – not looking like one, being one.

Anyway it buys him time. He could easily throw up. The last time he felt like this was when he did his Grade 4 bassoon exam when he was thirteen, fourteen. Bassoon. Not his idea, a pushy music teacher who took it upon herself to better his life prospects – everyone wants to be a pianist or violinist or cellist, but not so many bassoonists. There's more chance of getting into an orchestra that way, she said; imagine a boy from round here getting into an orchestra. But he failed his Grade 4 twice, passed it the third time, just, and gave up.

It's the same feeling of nausea now; not just nerves but the feeling of acting a role that isn't his, of not being himself. But then, that makes it easier in a way. He can convince himself that it isn't him doing it.

It's moderately busy in the shopping centre, but they hoped for that. Up on his right is the surveillance camera that monitors the entrance; he knows from years of looking at surveillance screens that there's a blind spot just below the camera, so he aims there, the narrowest sliver of space. He sees it, the cash machine, straight away, over on the left, as if it's the biggest, brightest thing in the whole place – as if it's the only thing. Someone's using it. He goes to stand in the queue, not looking around to see where the others are. He knows they're there, Mul, Lenny and James's friend, Paul – they'll appear from the shifting pattern of people milling about; they'll appear. He knows that.

The woman using the machine takes ages. It spits her card out and she starts again with a different one, then she messes around with on-screen balances, indecision over how much to take out. He doesn't mean to look, he just doesn't know where else to put his attention. There's no camera at this machine, it's too old, which is one of the reasons they chose it. Behind him he can feel the other three get into line, he can sense them. The way they all appeared at once so that there's now a queue of four people, off-putting enough to send anyone else to the machine ten metres further down.

She's done, finally, and she stuffs her card and cash in a handbag that's overfull and unzipped, an invitation to the opportunistic, he thinks, and he wants to warn her to zip it up. He normally would. He's like that, people say – always looking out for everyone. When she's gone he steps forward and pretends to go to his wallet for his card. Behind him, Lenny will have made the call to James by now. Just pressed call, then ended it. And James will be starting to do whatever it is he does with his computer to make things happen. So it's a question of waiting, pretending to be doing something with the buttons, feigning frustration.

Must be almost a minute by now. He hears a voice, Mul's, in the queue behind him. *Hurry up, mate.* He turns. *Sorry, problem with my card*, he says, and seeing Mul there, and the other two, just a glimpse of them, is a wash of relief.

Of comradeship, he thinks, then wonders where the hell that word came from. Some woman who's contemplating joining the back of the line huffs and walks off.

Then the whirring starts and the flap opens, and out it comes. Twenties at first, at a dazzling rate. Anyway, it seems that to him. Dazzling, the way they come in a blur of lilac. The way the machine goes so out of its way to empty itself for him. He pincers his fingers at the hole to hold the notes as they come out, to form them into a little stack, then he scrolls the stack (deftly, he's practised) in the palm of his hand and transfers the first lot to the inner pocket of his jacket – smooth, that's the thing. No grabbing, no rushing. Calm and smooth like nothing's happening. Three stacks, four, five; they fall down through the cut pocket into the jacket lining; bags of room in there. Bags. Then the tens come, which means the machine's been bled dry of twenties.

He's transfixed. His fear's gone, and with it any sense of where he is. Time both stops and speeds up; he's there for seconds and for hours, months, years. He could stand forever and watch those notes deliver themselves up into his fingers. It feels like something beautiful, really beautiful and perfect, the fulfilment of a prayer. It's not even about the money. It's the feeling that everything is all right. That nothing could harm him.

Then it stops, the money stops, and he pockets the final stash. Is the machine empty, or did James make it stop? Anyway, it's done. Suddenly his legs are liquid beneath him and his ears go deaf, there's only white noise, and the blissful feeling has turned into something blank, then rapidly into adrenaline. His heart kicks up. He lingers a moment, then walks away.

———

Can I escape this? The sword hangs. There is nothing to put my mind at rest – every day presents a new threat: the night. Every night is a battle, most often lost, and any victory is one day long, until its challenger comes along: the next night. I'm frightened. I understand why people kill themselves, or break down. I understand the bleakness of a life. The desire is to be a child again, to trust, to be comforted into peace and wellness.

I'm not going to reassure you, you have to learn to stand on your own feet, you have to learn to change your thoughts.

Can't. Won't.

Must.

∞

Pressing nocturnal questions:

Why do so many programmes on TV have the word 'secret' in the title? *The Secret Lives of Dogs. The Secret Lives of Five Year Olds. The Secret History of Ireland. The Secret Life of the Zoo. Secrets of Underground Britain.* Not so very fucking secret are they, if every other programme is intent on airing them? I don't know how it can be that nobody at the BBC or at ITV understands the meaning of the word 'secret'. Is a dog keeping its inner life a secret from us? Does it go around chortling conspiratorially to itself, trying to evade understanding? Is Ireland doing that? Is the zoo?

Dear BBC, They are not secrets, just things we don't necessarily know much about. I'll withhold my licence fee until you can clear up this distinction.

Why do so many TV programmes have 'Britain' or 'British' in the title? *How the Victorians Built Britain. Great*

British Bridges. Great British Bake Off. King Arthur's Britain: the Truth Unearthed. Brit Cops. Romancing the Stone: the Golden Ages of British Sculpture. Hidden Histories: Britain's Oldest Family Businesses. The Great British Sewing Bee. Secrets of Underground Britain. We get it. We live in Britain. Great Britain. Great British Britain. We get it.

Why is Brexit called Brexit, when it isn't Britain leaving the EU, it's the UK? Why isn't it called Ukexit? Never trust something that's inaccurately labelled. Even the name of this con is a con. Even the name is a shitshow, an almighty, extravagant, eternal show of shit.

Why have I started writing this story about the man who robs a cash machine and loses his wedding ring? This man who sprang to mind as an example sentence about recursion. Where did he come from – in what fissure of my cranium has he been concealed? Can you rob a cash machine and get away with it? Does he get away with it? Would he really do it, this harmless, decent man who's inherited my dad's love of David Bowie, this man who looks like one of my dad's old friends? Isn't it pushing credibility? He doesn't even have a name.

Is the story *going* anywhere?

Why are caravans called things like Pegasus, Sprite, Unicorn? Never a less sprightly thing did I ever see than the great off-cube of a caravan wobbling unaerodynamically along the slow lane on its tiny narrow wheels. It's like calling a shopping trolley Icarus, Voyager, Swallow.

∞

My stepdad's last day out in the world was spent walking by the sea and in a marine forest in Ireland. It wasn't his last day on earth, but it was the last time he saw anything of the world beyond a hospital room. Where he and my mum walked, there are white sand beaches with black, orange and grey granite outcroppings; the ocean washes in and out of deep peninsulas and estuaries, and the beaches give way to dunes which give way to a forest deep in ferns, mosses, ancient calcified roots of trees and the smell of pine.

This is what my stepdad saw that day. His last lungfuls of outside air couldn't have been fresher. It was late May in the north-west tip of Ireland, the land was luminous with near-perpetual daylight. He watched the roaring Atlantic. Then later that evening, back in my grandparents' cottage, he said he thought he was coming down with a cold, maybe flu. My mum went out to get him Beechams Powders, which he believed could cure anything. Later that night an ambulance was called. Two weeks later, after the intensive care wards of two different hospitals, he died.

My cousin's last day was spent out on his bike, a seventy-mile ride on a Saturday morning. He did the ride alone, and nobody had any contact with him after that. At some time in the next twenty-four hours he died, and his body was found by the police on Monday morning when his employer called them, worried because he hadn't turned up for work. He always turned up for work.

I would wish for my last day to involve an act of freedom – a walk by the ocean, a long bike ride, something I love. I hope that the walk and the bike ride were suffused with joy, with pleasure, for my stepdad and my cousin. Neither knew it was their last time to do that thing. If they'd known, would they have enjoyed it more or less? Eventually, everything has to be done for the final time. There must be many things that, without our realising it, already fall into that category for all of us.

Final acts acquire holiness. My stepdad's walk that day has. When we go to Ireland we almost always take the same route. We look out on the sea because it's the last sea he saw. We write his name in the sand. We reflect, each of us inwardly, that one day we will never see this place again either. It's a dull shock.

If finality makes something holy then every moment is holy, because every moment could be the last. That's a thought we spend too cheaply. Live each day as if it's your last, we think, and then we don't.

Everything is holy. It's only when we die that the holiness is called up. But it was always holy, all along.

∞

4 a.m.:

Then into the cocoon of that warm moment a thought appears and begins to open: don't think, it says. Don't think.

A voice in my head, which might be my own voice, my inner voice (but might not), dishes up the Larkin.

The million-petalled flower of being here.

The million-petalled flower of being here.

As if it could act as an incantation to sleep, or as my side of a deal that mustn't be broken – the Larkin poem had opened me and given me peace, and if I give the world my willingness, patience and peace, it should give me sleep. Shouldn't it?

Insomnia has turned me into a haggler. I'm always looking for the next thing I can trade with it or the next thing I can get from it, or the next bit of leverage I can use to cut a deal. When none of that works, it turns me into a beggar. I find myself pleading with it in the hope it will grant me what I want, when why would it? How could it? How could insomnia grant sleep? Isn't insomnia the very last thing in the world to plead to for sleep?

Whatever peace had been there has now diminished. Lie still, don't move. Often this feeling: if I'm quiet and motionless sleep might sneak in. Where did this thought originate? When did it begin to seem that sleep wasn't my right and could only be acquired on the sly, like contraband?

Then the thought: stop thinking. You are always thinking.

Then the thought: that was a thought, the thought to stop thinking.

Then the thought: that was a thought, the thought that it was a thought to stop thinking.

Then the reprimand: stop thinking.

Then the thought: was *that* a thought, or an order from my higher mind?

The thought: you think you have a higher mind?

Thought: I'm awake.

I turn over in a bid to start again. I'm angry with myself. Where did Larkin go? Where is my million-petalled flower of being here? The just-after-four flight from Bristol airport passes over in a distant smear of sound. I feel, suddenly, wide awake. Head abuzz on a slumbering body.

I switch on the light, get my laptop and Google I AM AWAKE. I don't know what I expect Google to do about this. The majority of results it returns are anyway about Buddhism whose blissful understanding of awakeness could not have been conceived by an insomniac. So instead I turn my raving, ranging mind to that vengeful little almond burrowed deep in my brain, the culprit of culprits, the amygdala, of which my hypnotherapist today did a crude drawing which set it at the centre of a page of multifaceted woe.

An article explains how fear and anxiety, often conflated, belong to different parts of the amygdala – fear arises in its central nucleus, which is responsible for sending messages to the body to prepare a short-term response – run, freeze, fight – whereas anxiety arises in the area responsible for emotions, a part which affects longer-term behavioural change. Fear is a response to a threat, anxiety a response to a perceived threat – the difference between preparing to escape a saber-tooth tiger that is here and now in front of you (because it's always saber-tooth tigers in the examples) and preparing to escape the idea of a saber-tooth tiger *in case* one appears around the next bend. While fear will quickly resolve – you will run away, fight it or be eaten – anxiety has no such resolution. You will need to stand guard in case, in case. Forever in case. Standing guard will make the perceived threat seem more real, which necessitates a more vigilant standing guard. Fear ends when the threat is gone, while anxiety, operating in a hall of mirrors, self-perpetuates. As a friend once said to me: there is no grace for the imagination. You cannot be saved from an assailant that doesn't exist.

For me, now, a puzzle emerges. What, then, fuels insomnia – fear or anxiety? Anxiety, everyone says. Anxiety, my hypnotherapist says; you are safe in your bed yet your heart is racing as if a tiger is present. You must learn to see that there is no tiger.

But there *is* a tiger: sleep deprivation. Sleep deprivation isn't a perceived threat but a real one, like thirst or starvation. It is the *fear* of not sleeping that raises the heart rate and tenses the muscles; fear, not anxiety. Here is where insomnia becomes intractable, because it deploys fear to act like anxiety. Where fear is a response to an external threat, insomnia is almost unique in giving rise to a fear that then causes the external threat. Being afraid of the saber-tooth tiger is what makes the tiger keep coming back – not seem to come back, but in fact come back. It is no use to say 'don't be afraid'. There is a tiger in your bedroom, you ought to be afraid. But it's not a tiger you can ever overcome by freezing, fighting or running from, so all your mechanisms for dealing with a real threat fail, giving rise to more fear, which keeps the tiger coming back. A vicious circle of Euclidean perfection.

The urge to take a sleeping pill suddenly overwhelms me; to be free of thought, of amygdalas and tigers. Well gone four, too late to take a pill – they don't work when it's this late, when I'm adrenalised with fear. Besides, I take too many; they give you cancer, dementia, so they say. I am exhausted to my marrow and down to the tip of each nerve ending. I lie down again with the light off and see myself being chased through a forest in the dark, my skin cut and bruised from multiple falls. Running, running. Running from what, exactly? What *exactly*? Death, I suppose, where every path of fear ends if you follow it far enough. The single-petalled flower of not being here, which bloomed in every one of our cells the very moment we were born. My heart doesn't thrup-thrup like it did at the beginning of the night; now it's a more lumbering, fatigued beat and the muscles in my chest and around my underarms are sore. Running from what? What would it be to turn around and face it?

So I turn, and stand. There's something there but it can't be fathomed and I don't know the word for it. Some sort of invisible force as if that little death-charge in my cells is being magnetised to a force outside of me; there's a sensation of static. I feel terribly small. Then the force takes form and becomes a red glow in the sky and assumes a spidery alien shape, and I realise to my dismay that it's the malevolent force in the Netflix series *Stranger Things*. In my most earnest attempt at understanding and confrontation, this is all my imagination can come up with, a hammy schlock-horror image of apocalyptic fire and alien invasion.

I begin to wonder if the makers of *Stranger Things* intended the series to be a metaphor for insomnia – the dark monotone world that is on the other side of this one, and the monster there that awaits you, a monster you must stare down. It will be getting on for 5 a.m. by now; I do a quick summary of which of the coming day's plans I can get away with cancelling. Panic wells. Those demons from the beginning of the night, until now merely lurking, are beginning to close ranks. I see now that when I write about those demons they seem to be a glib and lazy metaphor, but I do in fact feel there are demons and I do feel their advance, only that I know they are elaborations of my own psyche. They are an act of internal sabotage, the mind's attempt to rationalise and have control over a fearful outcome by bringing the outcome about. They're no less real for that; they're all the more real for that. And I feel them coming, and feel powerless to hold them off.

When I was a child I went through a time of having tantrums that were self-fuelled and increasingly senseless and went on for hours. I remember sitting at the top of the stairs beside myself with nebulous anguish, wishing somebody would come and make me stop.

My problem is that I always want somebody to come and rescue me. I am a coward. I have always been.

∞

Tennessee, standing in the shade in a steep, bouldered park, a clump of orange lilies on an outcropping, insects fizzing in the June heat.

My friend tells me about a man in her neighbourhood who gave up his lifelong Buddhism when a skiing accident left him with an anger he didn't think he should feel. All his life he'd practised the craft of Zen, of responding with equanimity and compassion. Yet the moment somebody skied into him, his response was rage and blame. So he gave up being a Buddhist and turned instead to God.

I picture a little handbook called 'Why Buddhists Shouldn't Ski'. *In general it is better for Buddhists to limit themselves to warm-weather sports and pastimes, the more sedentary the better. There is a reason why the Buddha is most often seen sitting. He was never found in the Rockies trying to outwit gravity.*

'Why, though?' I ask. 'Why would he give up a life-long belief for one bit of bad luck?'

'Because of his anger,' my friend said. 'Because all he felt was anger.'

'But no Buddhist I ever met said you're not allowed to feel anger.'

'Imagine you spend your whole life honing your mind so that when trouble comes you can respond without conditioning, respond without a kneejerk reaction. You know? Unthinking reaction. That's what he did, he spent his whole life trying to respond from a truer place in himself. Then, when trouble came, what did he do? He went straight to his conditioning. Anger, blame. Not truth.'

'What if the truest place in him at that moment was angry?'

'He wanted more for himself than that.'

'Why? He wanted more for himself than to be a human feeling human things?'

'Yes – yes. He wanted more than to always be trapped by the smallness of human things.'

'So he turned to God.'

'So he turned to God.'

My friend and I can't talk for more than six minutes before we get into the deep-and-meaningfuls. Small talk isn't in our chemistry. For a while we wonder at the beauty of this little place, our grassy plateau, then the drop into the woody glade. It's so hot. My friend lives on a mountain up above a city, a mountain partitioned and landscaped into dignified homes with preened lawns, pillared porches, verandas, coloured stucco. Cardinals flash red between maples. At dusk fireflies are floating embers in the darkness that collects between trees. Xibipiio-ing across the threshold of experience, here, gone. My friend has God. Whatever vanishes for her is held in the permanence that is Him. All of her steep, giddy drops have a landing place: Him. All of her belly-turning leaps are met with His open arms. All of her ecstatic soaring enjoys the safety of His tether. All the stale and eventless stretches of her life open into the wild drama of His love. My friend, standing here next to me, has all this, crowding her blood and bones in this moment, inflating her heart.

'There's a Buddhist image,' I say, 'it's a mural of a snake, huge, lunging out of flames, and on the end of its forked tongue, a monk meditating. It isn't about peace, a quiet life, not feeling things, not experiencing things. It's about the shit hitting the fan, and having the courage to sit with yourself, not hide, not deny – to observe the tumult from the end of the snake's tongue.'

'But for me, God is there too,' says my friend. 'That's the difference.'

Her once-Buddhist friend realised, she said, that he was fed up with doing it all himself. Buddhism is lonely, a solitary struggle with yourself with the hope of nothing except the eventual aim of no longer being a self at all. Obliteration of one's self out of being. All your struggle, just for that. All your years of trying to be a better self, only to be rewarded with that self's extinction.

And then it dawns on you that help is at hand. Far from being abandoned mid-piste with your broken ski, a fractured rib and a life's worth of anger, you find yourself in company, not only forgiven for your anger, guided through desperation, pain, disturbance, but also safeguarded from non-existence. God is there with you on the tip of the snake's tongue, on the cold of the slope, through the pain of illness, through the anguish of dilemma. He delivers a blossoming of being in life and after death – a process of becoming ever more gloriously yourself. A process of becoming ever-more, she said.

How can I describe this feeling I have when I lie down to sleep and it's as if I'm falling from a fifty-storey building, and there's nobody, nothing, to catch me? See, that isn't describing it. That's describing something else – falling from a fifty-storey building with nobody to catch me. What use is there in coming up with a metaphor of something I've never experienced to describe something I often experience? How can I describe the sense that underscores my life – all life as I see it – that nothing is known? Nothing is inherently certain. Everything is bottomless. How can I get to the heart of that?

You see, already the building metaphor doesn't even work as a metaphor, let alone as some literal evocation of falling. With the fifty-storey building the fear, presumably, is in hitting the ground, when really my fear is that there *is* no ground. I heard somebody describe his abiding anxiety as that moment when you tip back in a chair and think you're going to fall. That moment, but all the time. It's that kind of thing – that tipping point. It's not even about what's going to happen next, it's just the vertigo of the moment, when all sturdiness falls away.

Standing on this solid mountain of limestone on the border of Georgia and Tennessee, I envy my friend even as I try to argue with her. I can't make myself believe in God, not because of cynicism or some haughty deference to science, but because God is sturdy, a form of certainty to a believer, and I'm constitutionally incapable of accepting certainty. My mind can only see the provisional, never the incontrovertible. I can't help it. I'd like to help it but I can't.

We know that this table I lean on now isn't solid at all but a mass of floating atoms that has no edge. We know that once we get down to the atomic level of things we don't know, can't measure and can't predict very much. At its deepest reaches, experimental science becomes theoretical, abstracting from known observations and data to build explanatory models. Theoretical physicists are as much philosophers as scientists; amid the elasticity of their thinking is the central tenet: I do not know.

I don't mean to use pop-science to make a point. What do I know about any of this? I just see no evidence to believe in anything in the world except at a provisional and expedient level. And yes, to believe in things at a provisional and expedient level all the time, almost every moment of my waking life – but to accept that's all it is: provisional and expedient, not absolute, not certain.

One evening I was sitting in the pub with my sculpture group, a Wednesday evening; there was conversation which ran along usual lines – the project we were working on, the model we were sculpting, a lament at the state of the world, a rapture at some exhibition someone had seen, garrulous disagreement about what we ought to do next in the class. I was sitting on a stool. I suddenly felt that the whole thing was unreal. It crossed my mind that this scene I found myself in with these people in this pub might be a dream, or a hallucination stimulated by the prodding of some part of a brain in another dimension – my brain, my brain floating in some fluid somewhere, or my comatose body in a lab elsewhere in space and time, and the great solid solace of this pub, these people, was nothing. It was without substance. And these people, while seeming to constitute a safeguard against loneliness and isolation, were only synaptic notions produced by my disembodied brain, and were in fact proof of my isolation.

When I look back I think this was shortly before my insomnia started. I felt ungrounded in the extreme. I was often frightened. My mind was trying to think its way into stability and was finding only an edgeless expanse. What is real? What can I cling to? What can I rely on? I was always a worrier, but I didn't used to be anxious in this way. Worry is sensible to an extent, it has a practical dimension. I can't understand the advice so often given: no point worrying about things that are out of your control. Of course there's a point in worrying about these things. They are *exactly* the things to worry about; worrying about the things that are in your control is less practical since, instead of worrying, you could be doing something about them.

Worry and anxiety are not the same. Worry tends to be more temporary, more object-focused, more concrete, less diffuse than anxiety. Anxiety often has no object and transmutes itself into worry by finding objects to attach to, in order to justify its existence. This thing, this iterative, self-referencing battle with one's own thoughts, this is the strange being that is anxiety. I didn't used to have that, and now when I look back to that time in the pub, I can see that I'd reached a point at which anxiety had become so pervasive I couldn't perceive it was even there.

The problem with beginning to wonder if everything is a dream or simulation or illusion is that there's no proof either way. There's nothing in the world or in your own body, mind or brain that you can point to as proof that it is or isn't. In this sense, it's anxiety's jackpot. For me, the vertigo of it was terrifying; all my usual recourses to comfort were gone. What could I do? I could ask the person sitting next to me if he was real, and he'd say he was – of course he would. To himself, he could be nothing else. Everything in the world of the dream or simulation is programmed to believe in itself, otherwise the world would collapse. I could look inside myself for an answer, try to intuit or feel how something was as I'd done numberless times in my life, to feel the texture of things as they appeared to my mind, my trustworthy mind, my reliable heart, my logical brain. But no use consorting with my mind, heart and brain on the subject of their objective reality if they were a simulated mind, heart and brain that had been programmed to feel objective.

I see all this as indulgent, self-centred and a little mad. I also see it as a reasonable response to an anxiety that had become deep and persistent. Every comfort I looked to was failing me. Other people were, are, the ultimate comfort – in others there is fathomless solace; just in their presence. Not in their capacity to do or be or say anything, but in existing, a human shape in a doorway. This seems the same for other animals too – sheep will stay together in a field big enough for each to have its own territory, cows will gather in the same corner, horses don't like to be alone. Fish swim in shoals, birds fly in flocks. *Flock* is a lovely word. Originally *flocc*, and used only for humans – a group of humans living, moving and feeding together. Flock, also that softness of a tuft of wool or, once, a lock of hair.

And then this sensation, of tipping back in the chair and finding nobody and nothing there to catch the fall. Or more recently, the feeling is of too much energy in my head, of some frenzied current feeding up and out of my head, my heart racing as my energy is pulled upwards when all I want is to find ground under my feet. The ground rushes away. In fright, my mind looks for its flock, the soft solidity of others, and finds only uncertainty. The mind in fright starts turning in on itself, finding ways to frighten itself so that it can justify being scared.

Today an email arrives to my university address and it's from an Episcopalian priest in the US who writes to say that he has composed a Sunday sermon to give to his congregation that is, in part, about me.

He'd read my novel, *The Western Wind*, and was taken with it, so he looked me up online and found an essay I'd published about anxiety – about my anxiety and sleeplessness, but which then made a few wayward and tentative claims about anxiety in the Middle Ages. (This is one of the stranger aspects of being a writer, that people ask you to write essays about things and nobody seems to care that you don't know anything about writing essays, or about the subjects your essays deal with, or about anything, frankly. Anything. You make things up for a living and then you make things up in essays and nobody minds. Although, equally, nobody pays you.)

He sends me a copy of the sermon, this priest, and as I read it there is this displaced feeling I always get when a reader writes to me about my books. How can it be that I, here, dreamt up a world from some place in myself I can't quite name, and a person, there, has taken that world into a place in them that they can't quite name, and that unnamed place is moved and wants to convey it, and the conveying of it moves an unnamed place in me, and the echo passes back and forth.

That, and also, in this case, that this solitary and largely private nocturnal suffering of mine should be falling any Sunday now onto the ears of a congregation in North Carolina. In the sermon he talks about my novel, a little, and my essay, whose premise was that perhaps, *perhaps*, anxiety was less prevalent in the Middle Ages, given how many 'real' worries people had to contend with. He picks up on the sense of anxiety I describe, that of something groundless and objectless, something that has to find objects to attach to in order to maintain itself, but which originates without those objects. The mind inflates with a shapeless unease, he says. I find myself going over that phrase again, the loveliness of it, the aptness, the fact that shapeless is a word that occurs to me often lately: the shapeless dark, a shapeless fog of thought, the shapelessness of loneliness as opposed to that human shape in the doorway, the shapelessness of a life without sleep, where days merge unbounded.

He talks then about his own lifelong anxiety, there since childhood; his own shapeless unease. There is a caption in a scrapbook of his drawings and writing that reads, under a series of sketches, 'Aged 4. Tense, unhappy period' – that period, he says, continues into the present. This anxiety is given over to God; again and again he gives it over to God. And he petitions his congregation to think of Paul in Romans 8: 'Don't worry about anything, but in everything by prayer and supplication with thanksgiving let your requests be known to God.'

'The Lord is near' is the title of his sermon, and the words that precede Paul's exhortation against worry. The Lord is near. Don't worry about anything. In the Lord's nearness the priest finds a consolation of the highest and purest order, an opportunity to hand over his troubles without dwelling on or drowning in them, and to know that the opportunity is always there, since the Lord is always there. In this knowledge the world, he says, turns out not to be lonely and hostile as our tendencies towards fear would have us believe, but a 'sphere ruled by love'.

The Lord is near, he tells his congregation, with a certain humble surety.

Don't worry about anything.

The Lord is near.

I speak to another friend. He says science is the thing. The grand consolation. He quotes Clifford: *It is wrong always, everywhere and for everyone, to believe anything upon insufficient evidence.*

There is so much more evidence for the belief that we and the universe exist in physical form than there is evidence to the contrary. It's a question of critical mass; no single observation in itself could prove it, but the amassing of thousands, millions of observations that link together to form a set of conjectures that are verified and falsified and form a theory is something that begins to look robust, dependable.

For the theory as a whole to be wrong, so many of its component observations would have to be wrong. In the end, it makes far less sense to disbelieve it than to believe it. In the end you would have to resort to irrational thought to maintain a lack of belief in the objectivity of physical matter. You'd have to thwart the scientific process which has seen and proven the existence of all those building blocks that bring matter into being. Wide-eyed with wonder though science is, it is wonder at those things it's discovered, things it can barely believe itself, but which, like I said, it has more reason to believe than to disbelieve. Says my friend.

Reason, I say. Always that word: reason.

Reason, he says. Reason.

Reason versus faith.

Exactly, he says. Reason is the adherence to things that appear true by observation and experiment, not by a desire that they be true.

Truth. Desire. Here is William James:

> Our belief in truth itself, for instance, that there is a truth, and that our minds and it are made for each other, what is it but a passionate affirmation of desire, in which our social system backs us up? We want to have a truth; we want to believe that our experiments and studies and discussions must put us in a continually

better and better position towards it; and on
this line we agree to fight out our thinking
lives.

And on this line we agree to fight out our thinking lives. In
the pursuit of truth, which comes from nothing more than
a desire for truth, we fight it out. We think, says William
James, that 'there is a truth, and that our minds and it are
made for each other'. We think that the things we believe
must be pointing, not just at something believed, but
something believed because it is true. If all our beliefs point
in the direction of the physical world being real, then we
think it must be true, or we wouldn't believe it. We have
arrived at the belief using the tool of reason. Belief, reason,
truth. The mind's great trinity. So my friend thinks.

Do I feel consoled? Has my friend consoled me
with his belief in the monolith of reason? I don't feel
especially consoled. I'm wary of it. I can cling to the
titanic of science no more than I can cling to the titanic
of God. I don't see much opposition between science
and faith – isn't science just another form of faith – the
faith in reason? It struck me once that I can never be
faithless, I am always putting my faith in something –
be that agnosticism, atheism, violence, kindness, money,
cynicism, writing, love, politics, compassion. Faith is a

precondition for science, a precondition for everything. We must be willing to believe, else we wouldn't, and we must look for things to believe in, else we'd never find.

If a scientist tells me that light travels at 186,000 miles per second, I believe him because he believes it, and he believes it because he and other scientists have used experiments to verify the fact. But I have no way of measuring it for myself. If he tells me that, in theory, nothing can travel faster than light, I believe him. What else can I do? I can't check for myself. I believe him because he and other scientists have used theory to falsify and verify the fact. And what has brought him to have trust in his theories and experiments? His faith in reason as the basis for scientific enquiry. William James again: *Our faith is faith in someone else's faith, and in the greatest matters this is most the case.*

Religion is faith in a deity, science is faith in reason. The more I look at the two, the less difference I see between them. The more the believer in science holds up reason as the arbiter of all things, the more that reason starts to look like a god being worshipped. Reason is a thing that proves only itself. If you use reason to work out what is valid, you'll find that the only valid things are those you can reach by reason. These things we call 'reasonable'. So what? If you use God as the measure of what is valid, you'll find that the only valid things are those you can reach by God. These things we call 'godly'. This tells you nothing more about things in themselves, only about your process of arriving at them.

I think of my friend in Tennessee and the grounded way she walks, her feet slightly turned out, her runner's legs tanned and strong, and she is certain. She has what James calls 'a believing attitude'. God is like a lover to her, with all the passion, devotion and concern a lover provides, and an almost erotic power of presence. She is *his*. No matter how her mind strays she will always be his; she was born to be and will die being. When I lie in bed and feel the mattress and try to convince myself that the ground is rising up to meet me and that there's earth into which my roots go and that it's nothing, this hysteria which seems to spiral like an electric charge from the top of my head is nothing, then I want only to throw myself into some passionate and immovable belief, and I cannot.

And as the night struggles on one hour after another and I'm awake to see them all, awake and exhausted, I crave that feeling you get just before you go to sleep, when everything gives in. The fight ends. The fight of our thinking lives. Something bigger and stranger than yourself takes hold. Rest awaits. The relentless ticking clock of your conscious awareness prepares to be smothered, your limbs prepare to go slack, the things that hurt will stop hurting, the whole frenetic circus of it all is about to collapse. There's nothing for you to do, or work out. The priests and the scientists are made equal. They are made equal with the wild boar and the bat. There's nothing for you to assign your faith to but this one inevitable act of animal grace that is yours for the taking.

All the scientists in the world are looking for the beautiful order and logic that opens up in that silken path towards sleep. All the religions in the world were invented to express that mercy and grace that comes in the moments before we close our eyes, and go under.

∞

The insomniac is taking a swim.

She has a passable front crawl; it could be better but it gets her from end to end.

July. The sun is strung up near the top of the sky and blasts unEnglishly on a yellow meadow and a lake. The meadow grass is pierced with incisions intended for drainage – hard to believe when there's a drought and there doesn't appear to be a drop of water in the world. From above, even the lake doesn't seem wet. With the sun directly above it shines like a medal. And the parched grass is an old tatami mat, the drainage incisions are stitches in its fabric.

The insomniac is on drugs. A sedating antidepressant has brought her two nights of good sleep in a row and she's up, out, into the sun, swimming in a small lake in a meadow in Wiltshire. The sleep is normal, not the blunt anaesthetised dreamless coffin-like oblivion of sleeping pills, but a spacious sleep with dreams, and she's waking up bright, with bright thoughts, and energy that reminds her of how she was before.

Night three, night four, night five, she sleeps. She's there every day at the lake, a tiny speck from up here, going from jetty to jetty with propelling arms. One-two-three-four-breathe, one-two-three-four-breathe. There are so many layers of space between us and her, and all of that space is alive. Up here there's thin crisp air, and down a bit there's a cloud, just one, just hanging. Below that the birds, which are as big as her from this perspective – buzzards, pigeons, crows, magpies, swifts, all swimming at their own depths in the sky. Then there are the insects – the gnats, the midges, the mayflies, the banded demoiselles, the emperor dragonflies, the stone-flies, the mosquitoes, the net-wings. A swift plummets and plucks one off the water's surface just a foot in front of her windmilling right arm.

Everywhere, dragonflies, swifts. Dipping about in the air. Below the surface there are water fleas and nematodes and giant water bugs and scuds. Some small fish and tiny crustaceans. Even with goggles the insomniac can't see any of this through the water, which is the amber of brewed tea that's been lightly milked. She stops mid-lake to float on her back and look up at the dragonflies and swifts and magpies and buzzards and can find no words for how extraordinary the world is and how inexplicable and gracious is life; she can barely find the thoughts for it. From up here she's like a seed-head that's been wind scattered – pale, insubstantial, resilient and journeying. She goes from one end and back to the next, and then a lap around the three buoys before she gets out and sits on the bank. There's clay on her feet, it's good sculptable clay. The breeze rustling the dry leaves, and the distant clink and chatter from the café across the meadow and plenty of heat in the sun and so much of the day left. No *river shiver*, no *lake shake*. So warm, nothing to fight or overcome.

Night six, she sleeps, night seven too. She comes swimming. *This* is how the world used to feel, like there's space between her joints, like her thoughts aren't metal grinding against metal, like it isn't an effort to breathe; this clarity of mind and this lessening of fear and this feeling of possibility again. Like losing a disability, finding that you can walk again all of a sudden, or see again. Night eight, night nine, night ten.

In truth, the sleep doesn't come so convincingly now – a slight tolerance to the sedative already – but it comes and it's enough; she's used to very little and can make do. She must come swimming while she can and she must ride her bike and get on with work and get her mind straight while she can. We see her sometimes over in the café with a notebook, writing, writing. Night eleven comes, and nights twelve and thirteen.

She's swimming up and down. She can't help but see herself as if from above, because the thought is that there is something up there waiting to fall. The thought has been there since she began taking the drugs. What if they stop working? It's hard to trust in something so external and so apparently miraculous. She was brought up never to trust in drugs. Look outside yourself and you will fail. The cure for all illness is found in yourself. Have a cold? Meditate! Have a bladder infection?

Meditate! Have cancer? Meditate! Have a broken heart? Meditate! Up and down and then around the buoys, and swim as much as you can, she thinks, swim swim swim while you can.

Night fourteen is patchy; sleep comes but only after hours, and is gauzy. Night fifteen is the same. Never mind, keep going, it only has to last long enough to re-gain some trust and diffuse the terror. Every night is a small victory. Night sixteen there's little sleep and a panic attack. Never mind. Little sleep is still some sleep. She stops cycling to the lake and drives instead. As long as she can get in that water, which is the place of all freedoms and the antithesis of the dead dark night. She only has to hang on for long enough to outpace this. However fast the sedatives wear off, she'll gain strength and hope faster. Then she won't need the sedatives anyway.

From that imagined high vantage point, she's a swimming thing that's smaller than the buzzards, and she wonders if she could be small enough to go unno-ticed by the watcher. Or anyway, to not be worthwhile quarry. There is that line in *Tess of the d'Urbervilles* about the gods having finished their sport with Tess; maybe they've finished their sport with her too? She doesn't really know what the gods are; surely not malevolent beings, perhaps just an aggregation of forces – inner and outer – that have, over time, come to work against her. Bad luck? Why is it that bad luck feels so much like failure? Never mind, swim up there to that buoy and around the buoys and back, one-two-three-four-breathe, repeat.

Night seventeen, eighteen, nineteen, twenty; the sleepiness that used to come so quickly when she took the drug, and then came less quickly, now doesn't come at all. Zero-sleep nights are back, along with the routine panic. That levity in her limbs is gone and her joints feel clamped and sore and her head is a swarm of wasps. Keep swimming. It doesn't take much to get your head under water and move your arms and you must keep going. Don't give up on life. Affirm it. The dragonflies and swifts. Lie on your back and look up at them charging around. Glorious life, look at its speed and purpose, bombproof and beautiful.

From above, this pale starfished figure is like a piece of bait. She turns onto her front and crawls slowly end to end. It's brightish today but less hot and the water is darker and wind-chopped. There's panic between breaths and an illogical sense of being out at sea and alone and in danger. Stupid, there's no danger, it's just a lake in a meadow, she could stop swimming and float in half a minute to the edge. Stupid. But the sky is falling in. But it isn't falling in. She does another lap to prove how scared she isn't, and tells herself *how exhilarating! how brilliant! paradise!* when she comes up for breath. The breath a little snatched.

She thinks that we're watching her from above. We're not. We don't exist. She thinks there's an axe waiting to fall and that we wield it, but we've never seen an axe nor would we have any means of wielding one, since we don't exist. She gets out of the lake and dries off and feels the renewal of this pressure on her head, neck and shoulders which is the weight of whatever force has decided to crush her. Myself, she thinks. I am crushing myself. My doing. No heavenly forces. Any normal person can sleep; basic human function, not the work of gods. But that doesn't alleviate the pressure on her head, neck and shoulders, it only introduces a new pressure into her chest.

Never mind. Come back tomorrow. Try again. Night twenty-one, a little sleep, night twenty-two, zero sleep. The unbuffered days have piled on top of each other, her heart tries to beat itself free. Vague pain in kidneys. Walking across the hot meadow, a rapid shadow above makes her flinch and she covers her head – a buzzard flying at her. When she looks up there's no buzzard anywhere. She thinks we're out to get her, us above, eyeing her as prey. At the same time she knows we don't exist.

The chase and the defeat feel all the more crushing for being perpetrated by something non-existent. Never mind, swim. Head under water into the cool milky tea, up to the far buoy and round and back. From above she looks like one of those wind-up toys for children. She feels sorry for herself and cross at herself for feeling sorry for herself. There are still the dragonflies and swifts, and on the rushes and grasses by the bank there are countless blue damselflies; the swifts have come from Africa to be here. Someone's dog is flying along the lakeside, its feet not appearing to touch the ground.

Night twenty-three, night twenty-four. The world gets drier and drier. Every time she goes back to the lake she wonders if it'll still be there. Everything screams for rain. And yet the lake awaits, always awaits in its little meadow. Swim, swim, regardless. It doesn't take much to mill your arms and rock your body and kick your feet, the water does the hardest part. Head under, one-two-three-four-breathe.

∞

I haven't slept since Sunday night, I say.

I say this only after I have managed to dig my head out of my hands where it fell the moment I sat down. I have never cried in front of a doctor before, but there she was, straight backed, prim and discouraging. And I, unslept since Sunday night. Today is Friday. I can think of nothing but sleep. I would kill somebody if it meant I could have theirs.

This is a surprise, she said, and I sat and cried. Is it a surprise? I wanted to ask. She meant: you were only here on Monday. With her blessing, I've taken myself off the sedating antidepressants given that I'm not depressed (sleep-deprived, desperate, mad, but not depressed) and they're not sedating me any more. Since then, Monday, I haven't slept. Four nights in a row without sleep. I have looked on the internet to see if rebound insomnia is an effect of coming off them, which it is. The advice is to do it gradually, not at once. That wasn't her advice. Thus, here I am, once again a child with folded hands. This time a child in tears.

I need some sleeping pills, I say. She stares at me as if my tears have appalled her, or somehow confused her. Please, I say. Instantly I regret this because now the power is with her; now my night's sleep is a favour she can grant. And yet it is. And if it would help to fall at her feet and supplicate myself, I would.

Her face is stony, her demeanour sphinx-like. She hands me a prescription of fourteen pills; she offers no advice, no support. I take the prescription from her and leave without a word.

There's a metaphor I heard a long time ago when I was a philosophy student: an actress is on stage in a theatre when she sees a fire in the wings. She tells the audience there's a fire and that they must get out. The audience thinks this is part of the play and they ignore her instruction. The more animated and urgent she becomes, the more delighted they are by her passionate and brilliant acting. There's nothing she can do to speak beyond her role as an actress; every attempt only affirms the role.

I think this metaphor was part of a feminism course, but its wider resonance has never left me. Its relevance to life often applies. Here and now, in the eyes of the doctor, I am just neurotic and self-obsessed. The more I do to be listened to as a human being, the more I strengthen my role as neurotic and self-obsessed. The less she listens to me the more I tell or show her that I'm suffering. The more I tell or show her I'm suffering the more she thinks I am neurotic and self-obsessed. Each time, my role is reinforced and my role overrides my humanity. I become less human in her eyes. I am a type. I annoy her and waste her time, because all I need to do is sleep and I'm cured, whereas she has patients with real illnesses that can't be cured, certainly not with sleep.

No part of me wants to go to the doctor. I've come to dread it, to feel in it an absolute humiliation. I see her about insomnia as seldom as I can and when I go it is always for something specific; a prescription or, as before, a blood test. I know there's nothing in general a doctor can do. This time, almost four months after the last visit – a whole year now of having insomnia – I've come to ask for another blood test because I've seen a nutritionist who wants to check for any deficiencies, any thyroid problems, anything that might be contributing to my lack of sleep. The nutritionist is surprised that these tests haven't been run before. There's every chance that the tests will find nothing, but then at least I'll know. So I go in. I shake off the supplicant; a business transaction. I won't prevail on her for compassion or for understanding, I'll simply ask her for something practical she can give.

I wondered if it would be possible to have another blood test, I say. Everything I read about insomnia says you should rule out any underlying medical cause, and that hasn't been done. I know it's a long shot, but it would help me. Just to eliminate other causes would help me.

She turns to her computer and is silent. Finally, without any eye contact, she says, This is not a shop.

I look out of the tall sash window. A heron flaps steadily past above the canal. Rage and exhaustion are much the same sensation, I discover, a flame struggling out of the same dead fire. Anger is alive, energetic, object-oriented, but rage is what's left, eating itself alive. Rage and exhaustion eat me alive. They eat my deference, my past up to this moment, my future beyond this moment, my shoulds and shouldn'ts.

Now she is back-pedalling, as if she realises she has gone too far. But yes, she says (almost stammers), we'll do the test, yes, it's a good idea, let's do that. As she taps something out on her keyboard, I wonder if I'm in the presence of a maniac. Or am I the maniac? She has me in a game of cat and mouse and I don't know why. I watch the November sky, heavy and grey, and the pile drivers across the valley where new houses are being built. When I lived over there people objected to those houses; not me. I couldn't see the point since they'd be built anyway. Rage hollows my stomach, like driving too fast over a humpback bridge. Hands on my lap, primly linked, gentle hands. Not elegant but gentle. A lifetime of courting favours and having manners and asking nicely and never minding, never minding if the answer is no.

———

Radio 3; *The Women of Renaissance Ferrara*. It's lovely. It's just lovely. Those female voices in layers, he can't tell how many. With his eyes closed he can't imagine being anywhere but in a cathedral, even when he opens them it takes a while to believe in the sight of his kitchen.

The sun is hot on his right hand and thigh. His kids find it funny, him listening to Radio 3. Only people who live up on Woodlands Lane listen to Radio 3, his kids say, and anyway he's an old punk, that's what they think. It isn't true but let them think it, it makes him sound cooler than he is, or was. What he really liked was all those soft-metal bands that were around in the late 70s and 80s, with their ridiculous hair. He liked Rod Stewart; he'd never tell them that. And Kate Bush. His kids don't get Kate Bush. But maybe, he thinks, maybe there's something there in her songs that he can hear in the *Women of Renaissance Ferrara*, the way their voices take him somewhere else.

He turns the radio off when the doorbell rings. He lets Mul in and Mul sits at the half-oval of the kitchen table, in the sunlight, while he makes tea.

'Gail out?' Mul asks.

'She's taken Kelly into town to get – I don't know. Something-or-another.'

Mul nods. His look says all kinds of things at once. It says, Well she can afford it now, the something-or-another. It says, She's spending it already? It says, Does she know? But he knows she doesn't know, because that was the agreement between the five of them and it's set in stone.

'Jesus it's hot,' Mul says. 'Never known a summer like it.'

'You and Len going fishing later?'

'About three. You coming?'

'Gail wants to do something together. If you're going tomorrow I could.'

'Well, we'll see. Might do. We'll see.'

Mul looks older than his fifty-odd years; he looks tired, like he'd rather give it all up and fish for the rest of his life. They've each come away with a bit more than £13,000, which isn't enough to give it all up but maybe Mul can have a few holidays to break up the monotony.

Len and Paul think they should have jack-potted more than three machines, they should have done one each, but it was him, Mul and James who vetoed that. Three was enough, every one of them had scared him shitless and still does. Mul too. Mul looked almost sad when he got his £13,000, as if it made his years of work look like a mug's game. Which it was – everything was a mug's game, including emptying cash machines. Because you scare yourself shitless and then you've got your £13,000, and then what? What are you going to do with it? How do you even spend it, a brick of twenties marked with serial numbers linked to a crime? James is going to buy Bitcoin with his, and thinks they all should, but none of them know what Bitcoin is. Thirteen grand will buy you three, that's all they know, and they're not going to spend thirteen grand on buying three of a thing James can't quite explain and that doesn't exist. How are you going to spend it, then, James wants to know. You don't, yet, that's the thing. You hide it and spend whatever else you've got first.

'I was thinking,' he says to Mul. 'You should have a couple of grand of my money.

Then you can, I don't know. Just. Have it. For whatever.'

'No way,' says Mul. 'Nope.'

'Come on. A holiday for Mary, now she's feeling better.'

Mul lifts his hands and lets them fall onto the table. A Vicks Inhaler falls over, the one Gail uses for her hay fever. 'I didn't even do anything. I just stood in a queue.'

'It's not like that.'

He's about to say how they were in it together, himself, Mul, Lenny, Paul and James. They were equal partners – except for James, who got £10k extra for being the brains, the technological know-how – and they all risked the same. If one of them got caught they'd all own up. He doesn't say any of it because they've agreed not to talk about it now it's done. Never to talk about it again. It's done.

'I don't want it,' Mul says. He raises and tilts his cup of tea slightly, which is a gesture of thanks and blunt refusal.

Anyway, they didn't risk the same – James risked far more, passing himself off as a technician and getting into that machine, putting the computer there. Really, James deserved a bigger cut of the money, and he feels like saying that to Mul too because it's been bothering him. But James seems happy with what he got and happy to have taken the risk, almost as if the risk gave him more pleasure than the money will.

Anyway it's done, it's done. Five days since the last one in that shopping centre and they're by no means in the clear, and talking about it, even in your own kitchen, is asking for trouble. The doors are open, the neighbours just on the other side of that fence.

After that they talk about nothing much. Mul always calls round on a Saturday morning for tea after he's taken Mary to her painting group. He didn't for a while, when Mary was ill, so now it feels less like a routine and more like a special thing, a thing to be thankful for. So when Mul leaves he gives him a sudden, almost aggressive hug, a lung-rattling slap on the back, and he feels Mul's hand pressed against the back of his head, like someone would if they were going to push your head violently down – but without the push. With a firm clenching of the fingers, really briefly, a sort of weird, awkward comfort.

/

He doesn't feel the same as Mul. To him, the money is a godsend. He knows exactly what he'll do with it. He'll give it to Gail – a twenty here, a tenner there – for the rest of his life. Their kids are already provided for, all sorted out in wills, but he's never been able to give Gail as much as he'd like. *As much as she'd like*, says Mul in his head. Same thing. What she wants is what he wants. The two things have been identical since the day he first saw her.

He's never been good with women; in general he has no idea what they want. But with Gail it's easy; she wants the things you can buy with money. Money is love. He can do that. She doesn't want things that other women want, like assurances and time and poetry and sixth sense, some premonition of what it is that's needed in any given moment. He knows what she needs and he gives it, and she gives what he needs in return.

Today he gave her a few twenties before she went out the door, without Kelly seeing. Twenties from his own bank account, now he can afford it, not from the stash, which James says isn't safe to put into circulation yet. Spend it on yourself, he said. That look. Of delight, of gratitude and love, of having what you want. That was the look the kids used to have when they were small and were opening their presents, and it cracked his heart open so wide that it's never gone back to being closed again. And it was the feeling he had when the machine was spewing out money, which is what made it feel right – that what he got from giving her the money, and what she got from getting it, were the same thing.

That machine in the shopping centre gave them £18,000 in five minutes. It wasn't James putting the brakes on, he emptied it. It was as much as he earned in a year, and it still didn't come near what the last machine gave them. They'd been lucky, they'd picked their machines well and at the right time of day. In any case *he* thinks it's lucky; James thinks it was all about good planning and guile, but a life has enough failed plans – some of them great ones – to know that luck has the final say. The fact that James has sailed through to his mid-forties without finding that out is all the proof you need. Luck is everything.

He can't believe he did it. He just can't believe it. And it's that disbelief that makes it all right and gives him an unrealistic calm about what could happen next if they're found out – because honestly some part of him believes he didn't do it. Then, when the other part of him steps in and reminds him he did, he can say the mantra to himself: victimless crime. You're not really a criminal if the crime is victimless. You're an opportunist, no different to an entrepreneur, James says. You're an opportunist.

More than anything, he wants to tell Gail – it's the kind of news story she would tell him. Eighteen thousand in five minutes, she'd say. *Eighteen thousand*. In fact he's been half expecting that she *will* tell him. She'll read about it in their local paper or something, he's thought.

He's avoided the paper, the news, all of it; James said he'd keep an eye and let them know if there seemed to be any trail, anything to worry about. So far it's been reported like the other ones, but there's nothing the police have on them. And the police – says James – might give the outward impression of caring but they're not going to waste their resources on catching bank robbers. Nobody likes banks. Victimless crime.

Except, what he wanted to tell Mul today and couldn't, was that at some point that morning, in the shopping centre, he lost his wedding ring. It's always been on the small side and his fingers had swollen a bit that morning in the heat so he took it off, and he put it in his wallet. All that messing with his wallet at the machine, and the pretence of trying to find his card – it must have fallen out then. When he'd left the shopping centre he'd gone to put it back on, it was because of feeling elated, and wanting to connect that feeling to Gail. And it wasn't there.

He can't tell the others, even though he should – if it's been found near the machine, covered in his DNA or whatever, surely it's game over? But aside from that, there's something else about its loss that distresses him, makes him feel small, or that he's failed. That ring is the one thing Gail has ever bought him – it's cheap, but it used up all her money at the time. What a joke, to have made £18,000 in five minutes, only to lose the one thing he really valued. He can't tell Gail. He's scared to for some reason. *Because she's scary*, Mul says. But she's not, she's just someone who's gone without, that's all. Losing money and things, or lack of money and things, terrifies her, upsets her, that's all.

But what can he do? He can hardly go to the lost property place at the shopping centre and say, I was just robbing the cash machine last week and I lost my wedding ring. He can't even go back to the shopping centre itself, or near it. For now anyway – maybe ever.

Proliferations of love. A phrase he heard earlier on Radio 3. He wasn't really listening, he never listens to the chat between songs. Not songs. *Pieces. Symphonies.* Whatever. He was sitting at the kitchen table after Gail and Kelly had gone out, and he was thinking of his mother polishing her silver candelabra. It was all she had of her old life, before she married his dad. It was out of place in that little council house.

He was thinking of that when they said something about *proliferations of love* on the radio, and the phrase caught him. He saw silver light everywhere for a second, maybe the fusing of the image of the candelabra and the phrase, which didn't make much sense to him but had a feeling, like music. It felt like Gail was somewhere in that silver light, an outline of her in her wedding dress.

Then the singing had started, *The Women of Renaissance Ferrara*, and he'd gone into that reverie, thinking he was in a cathedral. He was never usually a daydreamer. In the end the doorbell had rung and he'd had to shake his head before standing up and letting Mul in.

———

5 a.m.:

The collecting tide of the night gathers itself up into a wave. Can't do it, can't do it, can't cope, can't go on. Too many nights awake, too much darkness and loneliness, can't do it. Am downstairs without knowing it, pacing, lunatic, shaking, tugging at hair, wheeling about in search of true north. My true north appears in the living room, shocked and sleepy, takes my wrists in his hands, Sshh, it's all right, it's OK, everything is OK, it's all right. Wishing to scream, finding myself screaming. 'No' the only word the brain seems to remember,

no to everything,

no.

∞

The next day, listless, sore-eyed, sofa-bound, panic moving through me in slow, low waves. He says, And now I shall perform for you my famous Flamingo Dance.

Then begins an awkward strutting, one arm aloft, one behind, the shoulders dipping, knees bending, this odd willowy form moving across my field of vision and back again. You are absurd, I say. Something dark and demoralised in me doesn't want to be amused, and yet there it is, a bubble of mirth finding its way up through the murk of my innards, bursting quietly into laughter.

∞

My self is a self understood through fragments. My self is a scattered thing. I look in the mirror and I don't know myself much. I look at what I write and it's like being introduced to my soul. Every time for the first time, not always liking what I see.

I know myself in ciphers. I know I am bothered and fascinated by that candelabra of my mother's because it found its way into this book and then it found its way into a story within this book. I hadn't thought of that candelabra for thirty years; then I thought of the song 'The Windmills of Your Mind' and I saw it as if the two things came together, when in reality they might never have belonged together. Then this nameless bank robbery man who I just made up is suddenly sad about it, about my mother's candelabra. I know that when I loan a character I made up a piece of my own autobiography I am trying to understand that piece of autobiography, and maybe they will interpret it for me and maybe they won't. Do I understand it now? No. It doesn't come that easily. Writing is dreaming. Not all dreams can be interpreted, and anyway, not all interpretations are right. And anyway, not all interpretations are interesting. And anyway, the dream is the thing unto itself.

Writing is dreaming. I only discovered that a couple of years ago. It is lucid dreaming – the work of the subconscious that has a toe in the conscious, just enough to harness the dream's waywardness. I always heard it said that writing draws on the subconscious, but that isn't true. It *is* the subconscious, and it draws on the conscious.

In the dream the subconscious finds ways to articulate, dramatise, embody things that have happened in waking life, things that are weighing on us, feelings, fears and desires. The dream is startlingly creative and expressive in doing this; it never fumbles for a metaphor, it never struggles for detail, it never labours over the unnecessary. It realises the ineffable. I dream relatively often that I'm swimming in a pool that contains only an inch of water. Even when I realise it has only an inch of water – a realisation that takes longer than it reasonably should – I carry on swimming. When I capture the feeling of this dream it is something intimately known to me – a complex but specific compression of many feelings that I can't articulate, something to do with futility, despair, tenacity, and which no other metaphor could capture as perfectly. If I were writing and I were looking for a metaphor for that exact admixture of those exact feelings in those proportions, I would seize upon that metaphor and be glad of it.

So it is. Some days I write, and what I write comes straight up and out of the subconscious without the conscious mind's interference. All that sediment, some of it gold or gold-ish, pours through words.

My mind is a cacophony. It thinks useful thoughts, and for every useful thought it thinks another four hundred useless, repetitive ones, and of those useless, repetitive ones a significant number are toxic. Shoulds and shoudn'ts. Eviscerations of self. Eviscerations of others. Terrors. Regrets. Reprimands. Old arguments. All of it arrives to me as an unedited babble, a firework continually exploding and dissipating, exploding and dissipating. Unedited, unreadable and impossible to assimilate. Just this constant crackling and sparking and exploding of mind.

If the mind is a cacophony, the subconscious is silent theatre; here are the players from the conscious mind, the fears, the desires, the ought and ought-not, but they are whittled down to a core cast and they re-emerge in costume. They come with colour, substance, emotion, tone and musculature; they come as ciphers, symbols and distortions all pointing towards the essence of what I am, whatever that is. Whatever that is.

Shoulds and shoudn'ts. Eviscerations of self and judgement and fear and anger and regrets. The mind is a tyrant; telling you what you ought and ought not to have done, which is never what you did or didn't do. The mind is a ninja. None of this matters when I write because

136

there are no oughts or ought-nots and there isn't even much of a self. There seems to be a locus of awareness, there seem to be hands feeling their way across a small landscape of letters which, quite mysteriously, harness what happens in that ghostly awareness.

Writing has saved my life. In the last year, writing has been the next best thing to sleep. Sometimes a better thing than sleep. I am sane when I write, my nerves settle. I am sane, sane. I become happy. Nothing else matters when I write, even if what I write turns out to be bad. I proceed from some open and elusive subconscious formlessness roughly called 'me', definable only by being nothing and nowhere, just the silence in which shapes move. Then words. Words harnessing things. There is the comfort of organisation, of shepherding chaos, not trying to abolish it but shepherding it towards borders, taking away the problem of infinity and entropy. Proffering the illusion of completeness. And somehow, I start to see myself out there in the words I've made, out in their many worlds, scattered and free.

A phrase came to me one night from nowhere: *proliferations of love*. It keeps echoing through me and I don't know why, but it feels like a definition of writing. The mind throws out thoughts and beliefs in so many permutations and configurations and we are enslaved by it, by the output of our own minds. The mind is a prison. And when we write the noise is distilled and alchemised, and the self can find a way out, which I think is what love is – the escape of the self from the self.

∞

'Do you stay in bed when you're awake?'

'Sometimes I get up, it doesn't help. I feel angry about getting up. I don't want to be up, I want to be asleep. There's a big spider in the living room that comes out at night. I don't want to be in the living room with a big spider. I want to be asleep.'

'You shouldn't lie in bed awake. Have you heard of sleep hygiene?'

'Yes.'

'Sleep hygiene is all about making your sleep routine as calm and regular as possible – regular bedtimes and wake-up times, no computer or phone screens late at night.'

'Yes, I've heard about sleep hygiene.'

'Keep your room dark and quiet—'

'That's all very well but my room isn't dark or quiet, I live on a road, there's a street light shining straight into my bedroom, there's constant traffic.'

'Have you thought about a blackout blind?'

'I have one.'

'Blackout blinds are really worth thinking about. Earplugs?'

'Have I thought about earplugs?'

'If noise bothers you—'

'Maybe that's my problem, that I don't think enough about earplugs.'

'Also no lying in bed awake for more than twenty minutes – bed is just for sleep and intimacy. It isn't for lying awake. Don't eat too late in the evening, no alcohol, no caffeine after midday, cut out sugar, no hard exercise after 7 p.m., a nice warm bath before bed but not too hot and not too soon before bed, keep your room cool and ventilated.'

'I do these things, they don't help.'

'Over time, they will.'

'Over time they haven't. I feel unhelpable.'

'Nobody is unhelpable.'

'I am.'

'Nobody is.'

∞

Fifteen years ago, a homeless man in Australia took against me one night when I was walking home on my own, and he pummelled my head with an unidentifiable object while I, hands on head, scrambled – ill-advisedly, I can see that now – into a small clearing under some bushes. When he had finished pummelling my head he disappeared, and I ran out of the bushes towards a taxi rank which was the only source of help in a deserted little town.

Waiting for an ambulance, on a bench with my head in my hands, my hands filled with bright blood and blood soaked the lap of my jeans and dripped onto my shoes in a way I couldn't comprehend, because it was coming from my head and was the sort of quantity of blood that suggests death, yet I was alive.

At night, fifteen years on, I force myself to remember this. The supposition is that remembering something objectively bad and frightening might take my mind from the abstractions of anxiety, might alert my skittering heart to the good fortune of being safely in bed. Feeling for the long scars at the crown of my head might prompt me into self-care and away from the impulse to hit my head against a wall. Enough damage to one skull for a lifetime, enough. Go gently with that good head. Likewise with my hand whose bones have been pinned together with a metal skeleton. And maybe if I replay that memory I might find it, the thing, the source of malfunction that fifteen years later surfaces as sleeplessness. Maybe a fear of the dark, a residual feeling of threat, an anticipation of attack that keeps me on my guard?

But it yields nothing. It evades analysis. Instead, with each replay the memory of the attack itself becomes more distant and uninteresting, a mere story. Even immediately afterwards I failed to find it much more than a story. In the hospital they offered me counselling, which I took because I was friendless in Australia and it was company. You're bound to feel traumatised, they said, appraising my broken, reconstructed hand and bandaged head, and I earnestly tried to, but in the end had to admit I didn't. I was worried that I wouldn't be able to draw and paint again, and that I wouldn't be able to play tennis. I might have played tennis four times in my whole life previous to that, so it seemed an odd worry to have.

I feel, I said. I feel. I feel blank. That's normal, they said, to feel blank at first. That's part of trauma. No, I said, I feel. Not blank like that, blank as in white. I feel – white. I feel white.

Whenever I've thought of the attack since, this whiteness presides. I waited for my experience of it to turn grey or black, and now understand that it won't. It was there when I had to single out the man from a photo identity parade, and to my surprise I recognised him at once. It was there when they said he went to prison; just a whiteness. I couldn't find any judgement or aversion to him or to anything. There seemed in me what I suppose I could call a universal well-wishing. A little like an evening I once spent on ecstasy, staring peacefully at a bush. Everybody else danced, and I sat for five hours on a tiny bridge in a Japanese garden in sultry August heat, wishing a bush well.

The feeling is white like a sky whose cloud cover is evenly backlit by an invisible sun, bright white; not empty. It goes straight to the belly. Warm, white, constant. It won't be further quantified. It refuses to compromise its whiteness or to break up or explain itself. I long ago gave up trying to understand it. Well-wishing reaches it only part way. The only word I've ever been able to find that gets to its centre is love.

∞

A girl and a boy – cousins they are – are roaming around the back garden, done with crouching in the laurel bed staking out the enemy line, bored with thudding the ball into the Norwegian spruce, no longer seeing the point of laying worms out on the patio and waiting for robins, incapable, today, of knocking the stone off the fencepost with another stone from ten metres. They've run around the bright grassy paths of their granddad's vegetable beds too many times.

Let's play something else, they say, but are out of ideas and catapult a couple of snails over the garden wall with hazel twigs, somewhat listless, and sorry for the snails.

At that a tall figure appears in black with a scythe and says, I have a game.

Yeah?

Yeah. I won't tell you the rules, or what the aim of it is, but you have to play it anyway, and reside with the persistent feeling of playing it wrongly – though there are no rules and there is no aim – and when you have finished playing you will both die. OK?

Not really OK.

OK?

Not rea—

OK! Go, kids.

Off sloped the figure in black and the girl and boy, despite themselves, began to play the game for which there were no rules and no aim, because it seemed there was no choice. The sky, summery, thickened to autumn and thinned to winter and lifted into spring and spread into summer, and they played while that pattern repeated, until several years in, both of their now-ripened minds comprehended the notion of death in a way their green kid-minds never could have, and they wondered in unison, Was that death, who visited us that day? I'm sure now I think of it that I saw a scythe—

And the sun, from afar, warmed the boy's scarred cheek, and warmed the girl's scarred hands, and negated the question with its gloriousness.

It would be years before they, the boy and girl, with their now-wise minds, comprehended the sun in unison and realised it hadn't been wholly honest that other time, with its optimistic warming of faces and fingers. Wasn't the sun halfway through its ten-billion-year life? Didn't it warm us up because it's burning hydrogen and making helium, and isn't it going to run out of hydrogen at some point, and contract, and die?

Isn't its very affirmation of life just the dynamic process of death? asked the girl.

I feel pissed off and cheated, said the boy.

He went for seventy miles on his bike.

∞

Love, love, grief, all bundled up, your stepdad died suddenly, too young, in a wealth of pain, your two granddads, your nan, your uncle, your cousin, some friends of friends, some friends of family, five dogs, two cats, that's all, you've been lucky, luck, pain, love, grief, life, love, loss, bundled up as one, the miscarriages you had, pain, much of it physical, Christmas passing under a blanket, bundled up childlike.

A child no less no more, watching a table being turned in a cottage in Stratford, all chilly and dark and beamed and thatched. School trip, nobody to tell about the wringing of the insides and the rap-rap-rapping of death. School-trip death; would make the local papers. Later the blood and the shame and the reckoning with a sanitary towel, and bafflement at being just that morning a child then passing all of a sudden into a woman. Not ready, not ready! Stampeding down the stairs unreadily, TV on, watching *Dallas* in a rage.

Two dozen years later bundled up, more blood, life is blood blood blood, Christmas a grey smudge. Well, that's lost then. You weren't ready. No wonder. No maternal urge ever urged in you, no wonder it all slipped away what with your doubts, what with your fears. Brimful with self, no room for a new self, so much more you always needed than to be always needed by someone else; 'mother' a strange word, brings to mind a rock, don't want to be a rock but rather to move, to ebb or flow, don't want to burden another with life. Feel the weight of life. Too much at times, not enough at others, ups and downs, sting in the tail. Death. Don't want to make and love something that will die. So. Onwards and upwards, get writing, comfort in that, the infinity of words, you're piloting a plane, you can tilt the world.

A half dozen years on (counting your time as eggs are counted), you realise. A hoax! The whole lot, the whole sorry lot. The question itself was a hoax, a sham. Will you won't you? Can you can't you? Yesno. Ready or not? A sham, a shambles, it was never a choice, it was never your choice. What did you think was happening – all that time, body like that, hips, womb, that blood, what did you think? Every month for three dozen years, gathering yourself ready to house a life like someone packing their bags for a grand adventure.

Grit, is what you see, persistence is what it is; a voice has called for thirty years. No thanks, you say, but it wasn't asking. *No thanks!* There's you: a stampede of rage. There's you, a child no more no less at a table, the table of Shakespeare's future wife no more no less. There's you, grown up, tilting pilot of your own craft, what-you-thought-was-your-own-craft, airstruck, wordstruck; there's you thinking maybe your destiny, maybe your destiny wasn't to reproduce yourself but to somehow produce yourself, bring yourself forth in words. Maybe because your womanhood started in so Shakespearean a setting your destiny was words, not dummies and nappies and schoolbags?

Not a lofty feeling, that. More a hope. Daughter of a builder who can barely read or write. First book he ever read was the first book you wrote; a year of anguish is what it took him. The only books he's read since have been the other ones you wrote. Falteringly read with gritted teeth. Bowled over with love is what you are at the love this shows, and proud and scared is what he is, proud his daughter can write those things he doesn't understand, scared because he doesn't understand. Doesn't know how literature ever got into your bones, Findus Crispy Pancakes and boil-in-the-bag curries more in your bones, your reading fodder the *Sun*, dad averting gaze daily from breasts. How did you ever write a novel then five? There's you, twelve years old in Anne Hathaway's kitchen, tables turning, destiny revealed. Coming-of-age. Womanhood, adulthood is for making words not kids. That's what you came to think.

Five novels later. Come to think, what were you thinking? Words. Words! All that blood just for words? Didn't you notice? It's not a choice. Motherhood not a choice. It chose you, it was there when your two X chromosomes first showed up, nothing to do with Shakespeare or tables. Way back, thirteen years before, that's when. You turned down an unturndownable offer. Let your brain decide on what your body had already decided. Not your fault. Nobody prepares you.

Never got round to doing what everyone else was doing. Never managed to get a mobile phone, maybe will one day when everyone else has progressed to telepathy. Never could buy into it all – kudos of mothering, the bump, the blooming, the breastmilk, the birthdays, the boredom, the blessings. Mother nature, mother earth, virgin mother of Christ, mother of all. Mother. Never minding about all those dreams. Set them aside. Never mind about shaping your life, its shape is what's left, the negative space made by this new creation. Become a negative space, be eclipsed by your own light. That's what you thought. So you didn't.

Also thought overmuch of death, of dying, of leaving or being left. Extrapolated from love of nieces (fierce and deep) to love of own child (fiercer and surely tiger-like and unbearably hot to the touch). Then extrapolated from love to loss, as too often the case. Overthought. Life is hard. A strange gift. Oft-unkind gift. Not my right to be the giver, to make such a choice. Not my right, you thought. So life said: Who'll give me then? If not your right then whose? Not my right, you answered. Fair and stubborn like you are.

Time elapsed.

What, then, will you do with this wash left by a gone-out tide? What's here? Words. The past, corpses strung up in a row. Sleepless nights. A dog barking. A walnut tree shrugging off summer. A morning mist. A white, bright sky, not empty. A white feeling. Surfeit of white, the double kiss of your female chromosome, underused, overspilt, the wash of a gone-out tide.

A choice, you thought. A take-it-or-leave-it? Not your fault, you weren't to know. Can't leave what's gene-bred, can't leave yourself. Watch. Your own tide going out. White sky is what's left. So bright, as if backlit. What will you do now with all that? That white? For-want-of-a-better-word-love. Love, grief, loss, love, life, love, all bundled up. Irrefusable. Now. So much of it, hands full, not enough places to pour it. You refused the irrefusable. So now what will you do?

∞

'Why don't you spray some lavender on your pillow?'

'Because I'm beyond lavender.'

'It can't hurt to try.'

'It can't hurt to rub myself down with dry beech leaves in the moonlight, but will it help, is the question.'

'This is all about staying positive.'

'Is it?'

'No spirals of negative thought. It might sound like an old wives' tale, but a hot milky drink at bedtime does help. Nice comforting things, little acts of kindness towards yourself.'

'Does jumping out of a top-floor window count as a little act of kindness towards myself?'

'Are these sessions helping, would you say?'

'Yes.'

'So, try the lavender. And stay positive, and focused. Remember, no staying in bed awake. Get up and do something unchallenging. Unload the dishwasher. Do some ironing. A jigsaw puzzle perhaps. Nice and gentle. Yes?'

∞

I don't have a dishwasher, or an iron. I once had an iron but I don't know where it is any more.

Tower of London Remembrance; an expanse of poppies cascades impossibly from a tree and over a wall, into a lake of red. There's a fictional London skyline behind.

£4.99 from Save the Children, which is quite expensive for a charity shop puzzle but the expanse of indistinguishable red appealed to me. It spoke of the passing of many small fruitless hours. With the humble and obedient fortitude of someone pious – Margery Kempe or Julian of Norwich – I set myself out on the living-room floor at 2.30 a.m. with the back of a painting as a board and fished through the five hundred pieces to find edges. Red edges down here, grey-blue up there. Surely not enough edges; nowhere near enough.

Tower of London Remembrance is a wooden puzzle with a few novelty pieces, all war-themed. A piece of puzzle in the shape of a rifle. Then another in the shape of a soldier, and one in the shape of a boot. A helmet. A tower. A horse. I didn't know my life would ever come to burying a boot-shaped puzzle piece in the Gherkin at 2.30 a.m. There are some moments of life that arrive as if they have nothing to do with me, like postcards falling on the doormat. I can watch myself living them. Their weirdness, or mundaneness.

3 a.m., 4 a.m., one night after the next, the sea of poppies comes together, and the night falls apart, and I take myself to bed at five or six. I feel low. The world's a bear pit, I think. All those men dead in trenches. We wear poppies and still go to war. The next night *By the*

Thames, a two-pack puzzle, comes together – one poorly painted tableau of Windsor Castle, and another poorly painted tableau of Marlow with a jetty, a bridge and an astonishingly unrealistic rainbow arcing over the church. Never enough edges, when you lay them out. And yet no cause for fear: the staff in Save the Children count the pieces of every donated puzzle to check they're all there.

With the lamp lit low and the snow coming down out in the blackness and the temperature in the living room reading fourteen degrees, I'm arrested by this act of care. Someone has counted these pieces. Someone unpaid has counted these pieces so that nobody will be disappointed; so there'll be less disappointment in the world. Maybe it's not a bear pit. I thread together the garish rainbow, the church spire, the bridge parapet. Marlow appears.

∞

Great British Bridges. The Great British Bake Off. The Great British People.

The Great British People have spoken!

Grammatical note: the 'great' in 'Great Britain' refers to the collection of nations that make up the country, as

Greater Manchester refers to the collection of metropolitan boroughs that make up the city. In as far as 'great' is an adjective here, it's one that means 'including adjacent areas', or 'combined' or 'large' – as in the Great Plains or the Great Barrier Reef. But lately that adjective has morphed subtly in meaning to its more subjective use of 'above average', 'most important', 'really good', 'excellent'.

This morphing of the word *great* is a subtle, gentle confusion, a little play on words that seems harmless. Then it's used in ways that evoke two very particular ideas of nationality – one that conjures an imperial virtuosity – *Great British Bridges, Great British Railway Journeys* – and another that conjures a wartime zeitgeist, an almost quaintly collective pulling together – *The Great British Bake Off, The Great British Sewing Bee, The Great British Allotment Challenge*. This is all very nice; why not celebrate our illustrious past, why not pull together? Why not celebrate ourselves as a nation of tea and gingham tablecloths and bunting and fox-glovey summer days and deep, sensible conservatism? Team Britain. Why not? It's innocent enough, and surely we should be allowed to have and celebrate a national identity.

But changing the meaning of the word 'great' is insidious. It gently touts the *Daily Mail* line of our grand old sighing nation, avuncular and nostalgic, superior, granting favours to its less great nieces and nephews. It's never clear what exactly the 'great' refers to – what deed or quality. Great at what? Great in what way? The echoes of the phrase *Great British* are of stature, standing, pride at best, pomposity at worst.

This might not be a new use of our country's name, but it's been used these last few years to the point of becoming a strapline, a brand. Great British Values, the Great British Public. These are straplines belonging to the rhetoric of David Cameron's Big Society government and frothed up by the right-wing press – an article in the *Telegraph* after the 2015 election that gave Cameron a clear win sported the headline: *The election's other winner? The great British Public.* (Hindsight makes this headline even more absurd than it was at the time.) *Great* here isn't capitalised; the *Telegraph* isn't even pretending that the word 'great' belongs to the country name Great Britain; it's just an adjective that describes it. The brilliant British People. The super British People.

I find this deeply strange, and deeply suspect. Who says we are great? *Great* meaning what, exactly? I ask again: great *at* what? At being British? At voting the way the *Telegraph* wanted us to vote? Great since when?

Always great, or quite recently? All of us? Or just the ones who voted the way the *Telegraph* wanted us to vote?

∞

I'm angry about death. I'm angry about factory farming. I'm angry about this family of Yemeni people who've been reduced in number and made homeless by the senseless machinations of war and alpha-male politics. I'm angry that my MP, the person who represents me in parliament, is Jacob Rees-Mogg. I'm angry about the heedless repetition of historical mistakes. I'm angry that the week we gained Donald Trump as a world leader we lost Leonard Cohen, in some deal that even the Devil must have flinched at. I'm angry that nobody obeys the speed limit through my village. I'm angry that nobody even obeys double the speed limit through my village. I'm angry about the great national con that is Brexit. The rip-off of our values. The insult to our nationhood, where by some horrible trick our self-assurance has been swapped for arrogance, our tolerance for superiority, our power for meanness, our natural trepidation for outright fear. The people are angry, they say. The people are hitting back.

It's true; the people *are* angry. This person is angry. And I know fear. I have seen more 4 a.m.s this last year than I can count and 4 a.m. is a time rife with fear. A car races through our village too fast, hits the speed bump outside our house, drops from it at such pace that our bed shakes and I'm awake. You fucker, I think. I bet you voted Leave. Then I want every speeding car, every over-entitled SUV hurtling through a 20-mph zone at 50 with Darling #1 and Darling #2 in the back and Spencer the Spaniel in the boot to be banned from my village, banned from polluting the air I have to breathe. Maybe we could give Leave voters Kent, I think. We could partition it off and they can have it.

The thought lends a rare deep hour of rest.

∞

6 a.m.:

The night is another planet a bit like our own. Dark, of course dark, but darkness is a hundred things coming by degrees, darkness is spilling around multiple points of light. The rectangular outline of street light around the blind. The clock on the oven that makes me cry with its painful reporting. 2.26. 3.49. 4.11. 5.48. The neon LED display of the homemade weather-forecasting gadget that colours the kitchen green and orange (coolish now, warmish tomorrow). The standby of the stereo. The flashing red of the monitor. The green of the battery charger. The night sky through the French doors and sometimes the moon turning the living room blue. The various blacknesses of the garden as it slopes away. The distant bulk of the hill opposite and car headlights winding down it in a steadier stream. A police light.

Tonight the moon has been a rich sumptuous yellow, a fat crescent, low as anything. And Jupiter by its side. Now I look for it, as a winter morning edges in, and it's on the other side of the sky, smaller, higher, but still surprisingly bright.

The garden table emits whitely from the patio, the copper beech is a giant emerging to the trained eye. I can imagine the grass and the borders and the acer in its pot, but can't see them. Is the garden in darkness or is darkness in the garden? Is darkness an appearance? A dark garden, like a blue coat. Is darkness a state? A dark garden, like a cold sea. Is darkness a quantity? A dark garden, like a full glass. Is darkness a judgement? A dark garden, like a difficult sum.

Beyond panic, and well beyond sleep, I sit on the sofa and watch as the day comes, grain by grain, like ash falling. Black things turn toneless grey. There emerges in the garden the things I know – the paving and the steps and the grass and the broken bench, the pile of branches from the cut-back hazel, the sculptures I made and never finished, the little cherry tree with its prayer flags. A square of greyish yellow, a square of ashen red.

Proliferations of love.

He sticks the headphones in his ears, he doesn't like those little earbud things but he's too old to wear the over-ear ones, his son says he looks like a dick in those. Which is probably true. He still has an old MP3 player which he insists on using because it's simple and it does one thing which is the thing it was made to do, not like phones which do two hundred things, none of which seem to involve phoning. His son's put 'Absolute Beginners' on the MP3 player, but that's all. That's as far as he got. So he listens to 'Absolute Beginners' all the way to the shopping centre, six times over.

The height of irony, really, that this fifty-two-year-old luddite should have just jackpotted three cash machines. Jackpotted. A good word, better than 'robbed', more innocent sounding. In truth he has no idea how it was done – how a computer a few miles away can control a computer in the machine. Even when he and James were growing up, James would do things with their Atari that were beyond his comprehension or interest, program it, code your own game. It beats him how James ever learned to do any of that, where the knowledge came from; not their parents. But it seemed to be in James's genes somewhere. That, and risk-taking – a kind of screw-it approach to everything.

I absolutely love you. He loves that line, absolutely loves it. His last act of freedom, if you like, was going to see Bowie in Berlin with James in 2002, when Gail was pregnant with their first, and it was like being dropped onto another planet for one night. There was no way of describing it when he got home, so he didn't. But he wished afterwards that he'd chosen 'Absolute Beginners' to play while Gail was walking up the aisle.

Imagine it, it's perfect really. *As long as we're together the rest can go to hell, I absolutely love you, but we're absolute beginners.* Perfect. Maybe he should marry her again just so he can make that happen. Though divorce is more likely on the cards if he doesn't find this ring – or, not divorce but something worse, silence, disappointment, a gradual soft killing of him because he's let her down.

He isn't going to find this ring. He doesn't even know what he's doing going back to look for it, as if it would still be lying there by the cash machine five days later. When he gets to the entrance of the shopping centre he can already see that it was a mistake; the machine has been taped off by the police, with a sign too far away to read but which must be asking for witnesses, and the sight of it makes him feel like throwing up again.

Just tell her you lost it, he thinks. So what?

Go back, you idiot. Go home.

/

She looks for a long time at something just past his ear. A really long time. The only part of his body that he's aware of is his ring finger which feels indecently naked, like that man on the beach at Dorset last summer. Gail hadn't been able to look and had sat, staring ahead and occasionally throwing small stones at her own feet. 'Why does he have to keep walking around all the time?' she said. It was true, he did a lot of walking around, that man. It was weird to see a man starkers like that, ambling up from the sea. No matter what, you could only see what was hanging between his legs, wherever you tried to look, that was all there was. Weird, because who cared? It was just an old man's dick. But it was somehow everywhere.

'I'd really like you to find it,' she says. 'It's our wedding ring.' Her gaze falls briefly to her own hands, but then lifts to stare past his ear again. Teary-eyed. 'Anyway.' She shrugs. Her shrug seems to say, *go on, fail me*. Then she shifts round and stands up from the bed and disappears to the bathroom.

It's just that it's always been too small, is what he said. That's why he has to take it off when it's hot, because he's scared that his fingers will swell and the ring will cut off his circulation. Nothing to do with him not loving her, just to do with it being a bit too small.

That was when she looked past his ear. 'Well, sorry about that,' she'd said. 'Next time I spend everything I have on you I'll try to be more thoughtful.'

That was when he'd failed her. Not in losing the ring, after all – she'd taken that pretty well – but in seeming to blame it on her. He lies down in bed. He hears her go downstairs and the TV go on; it's gone eleven. He's about to follow her down and make things up but suddenly he's thinking of that candelabra in the cabinet in the living room, not even on display – just at the back of the cupboard behind some unused place mats and a box of wallpaper paste that had never found its way out to the shed. He'd thought Gail would like that candelabra. When he said it had belonged to his mother she'd tried to look grateful but she'd put it straight in the back of the cupboard almost as if it disgusted her.

I absolutely love you.

There they are, the perfect words. I absolutely love you. For a while he listens to the half-comprehensible drone of the TV in case there's news and his *jackpotting* is on it. *Police think they've found evidence that might be connect-*

*ed to the robbery of a cash machine in the Chequers
Arcade last Tuesday.*

But there just seems to be the babble of a
sitcom.

/

Proliferations of love. Vows and confidences
and wedding bands, long nights up with the
children, years of devotion, doing your best.
Years of being stuck staring at surveillance
screens, him, Mul and Lenny, a quartet of
screens, nothing happening four times at once.
My husband works in security, Gail has been
known to say, and it's a phrase that's both
somehow bland and enigmatic at the same
time so that people tend not to ask more.

James is looking at him with a kind of tender judgement. 'Where've you gone?' he says.

'Nowhere.'

'Nowhere,' James smiles. 'Everyone is always going nowhere.'

'Meaning what?'

'Have you ever noticed that if you ask
someone where they've gone or what they're

thinking about, the answer is always nowhere. Nothing. And I believe it, that's the trouble. It's sad that we can do anything with our thoughts and instead we go nowhere and do nothing.'

His impulse is to reply, 'Actually it wasn't nowhere, I'd gone somewhere, I was thinking about escape.' But he can't decide if James is trying to bait him and wants him to admit something like that. Also, he's bothered by that word, escape. Was that really what he was thinking about?

'I want to do another one,' James says, and he marks the declaration by hurling a teaspoon of jam at his scone. 'Just us two. It's not worth anything if you split it five ways, but halves is worth it.'

That's it, right there – the way James eats his scone. His stupid bloody scone. He eats it as if it's a stupid bloody scone and as if it's the best thing mankind could eat, at the same time. It's like he realises how pointless everything in the world is, except things stop being pointless as soon as they're done or touched or eaten by him.

'No,' he says, just like Mul said to him a few days ago. 'No way.'

James just keeps eating. So he says it again: 'No way.'

The place is packed and noisy and one of those bullshit places that has people getting hammered at the bar on £9 pints of Belgian lager while off to the side others, like him and James, sit on plush seats at white-clothed tables by purposefully tarnished mirrors and have afternoon tea. £35 a head, is afternoon tea. He laughed out loud when he first walked in and went up to the table James was rising from, and James grinned as he does and hugged him lovingly as he always does.

'Well I've got the technician's outfit now,' James says, 'so I might as well get my money's worth out of it.'

'Don't you think you already have?'

'Come on. Think about it. All you have to do is stand there and let a cash machine empty its contents into your hand. That's all. I'll do the rest and we'll split it in equal halves.'

'I can't,' he says. 'How can I? I've got a family for Christ's sake.'

In response to which James elaborately pours them more tea, from a great, splashy height.

My husband works in security. He hates the phrase and wishes Gail wouldn't say it. It's not MI5, he's told her. I monitor an office block at night. Sometimes I monitor the car park. Mul and Mary long ago made a joke of it – Mary says Mul works in insecurity, given that security jobs never seem to last more than a few years; budgets get cut and security guards are the first to go, or their jobs are outsourced. You can look at a screen from anywhere. But Gail has never really had a sense of humour, not like that anyhow; she wouldn't be one to see the opportunity for a joke like that.

James sits back and says nothing. He has such a nice face, does James – all boy-next-door, slightly tanned honest goodness, and something really, truly kind in his eyes that can't be faked and can't be lost even as the years pile on.

He looks like their mother. Any sighting of James is a sighting of their mother, and also the opposite – a sighting of her disappearance,

166

if you can sight a disappearance. When she left, he had to look after James because James was eight years younger, so James – his strange devotion towards James and James's towards him – has become the same thing as their mother leaving. It's also the same thing as the silver candelabra and goblets given to her by her parents, which she polished whenever their dad had laid into her. And that she left, that she got fed up with being laid into and beaten up, was the evidence of a part of her that got handed down to James, not him. James walks away from strife, or doesn't get himself into it in the first place.

'D'you have any – qualms, about what we did?' he asks.

James's answer is immediate but thoughtful enough, as if he's already weighed it up and resolved it in his mind. 'No. Not even a bit. We're ripping off banks. Banks. They're ripping us off all the time. We, the taxpayers, paid for their folly when it all went tits up and they got away without a scratch. This is a small scratch, what we're doing, it's puny but it's something.'

'I still can't believe we did it. *I* did it.'

'Do it again,' says James.

He has an image of Gail looking past his ear, not at him. James is looking squarely at him, always does – whatever he's done or hasn't done, James still looks him in the eye.

What would he do with another fifteen, twenty grand? What could he buy for Gail or the kids that they don't already have or that would be appreciated without really going noticed? Too many hand-outs would start to look suspicious, and anyway, his life probably isn't long enough to spend it that way. He'd die with a small fortune in a lock-up on an industrial estate and the storage company would get it since nobody else knows it's there. He could leave it to James, but James doesn't need it. Or he could just run off with it. He wouldn't. But he could. In fact, that's the *only* thing he could do with it.

Proliferations of love, love which on occasions looks like servitude. More and more it looks like servitude these days. He doesn't like to think, doesn't like to think how much money he's given, then there's the time, then there's these cash machines and the stupid, monumental risks he's taken – not for himself.

Now, suddenly he's thinking. He's thinking of hills for some reason, not mountains but soft hills and thunderstorms and David Bowie on stage in Berlin with his hair fluttering and *The Women of Renaissance Ferrara* and a drum beat and twenties spewing from a cash machine and his mother by the window in their living room and James's undeniable smile and there's James in front of him now and looking at him feels like something rushing through him, a wind blowing open a multitude of doors. That's what it feels like. That all his doors have blown open.

He goes to speak and he suspects the word that'll come out is yes. Yes. I'll do it, is what he's going to say. Then his gaze follows James's, which has gone towards the bar where two policemen are talking to the bar staff. The policemen turn, then, and start scanning the room. The thing rushing in him keeps rushing, rushing. He feels for the bit of flesh where his wedding ring used to be and the doors that have flung open in him are

pinned back and the thing keeps rushing,
rushing.

———

7.30 a.m.:

Here is the pile of yesterday's clothes on the floor. I pick
them up. Or, if bedtime superstition corralled me into
folding them roughly and stuffing them in the cupboard,
then I take them out again and put them on the bed.

I get into them in the precise reverse order I vacated
them the night before: bra, top, jeans, jumper. Always,
something unbearable about this process – the process
of getting dressed in the morning after a night of no
sleep, getting into the very clothes you took off the night
before when you embarked on the ritual of bedtime as if
such things as sleep applied to you any more. The pile of
clothes is an open rebuke. I want to say they mock a lost
innocence even though I know this makes no sense, but
more and more I make this unconscious association between innocence and sleep.

I suppose it isn't a new association; it's one I made myself when I wrote that opening line in my novel: *I sleep
the sleep of angels*. It's one we make from childhood – the
sleeping infant, untroubled by conscience or the weight of

the world, or in the fairytales that have people slumbering for a hundred years or rendered inert through the petty evil of others' potions and spells; it's there in Shakespeare when he writes, in *Romeo and Juliet*, 'where care lodges, sleep will never lie', and in that line in *Macbeth*: 'innocent sleep, sleep that knits up the ravell'd sleave of care'. 'Balm of hurt minds', he calls it. 'Chief nourisher in life's feast'. And there it is in death, the ultimate surrender and eternal rest, the dreamless sleep, the reconciliation, the forgiving annihilation, the letting go no matter what. No matter what your life was, there comes this final benediction.

Sleep. Sleep. Like money, you only think about it when you have too little. Then you think about it all the time, and the less you have the more you think about it. It becomes the prism through which you see the world and nothing can exist except in relation to it.

In yesterday's clothes, I go outside and traipse up Solsbury Hill with overworked heart. This morning is grey but not dull. January light is unlike December's, already it has the beginnings of that clarity and expanse that culminates in spring. The snowdrops are little acts of resistance. The dogwoods are wine-red. The sloe bushes turn the hedgerows pale blue. Beautiful, surprising blue; a colour reserved more for water and sky, you don't see blue that much otherwise in nature. The hazel has a mass of ochre catkins hanging in busy vertical marks like they've been made by a typewriter. The branches of that tree there, whatever it is, are frilled with lichen that has its own inner sunlit luminosity. A dog tries to eat my scarf. The sun has just come up from behind the opposite hill and nudged open the grey, and now the hilltop is momentarily orange. Then gone again. I find myself crying.

What is it we're supposed to make of life? There is so much suffering – my own is a tiny stitch in a vast tapestry and many, many people suffer so much more than I have. What is it that keeps rising up in us even when we feel crushed? What keeps putting one foot in front of the other, or looks at the vague blue smudge of a sloe bush and is reminded of a truth that doesn't even have a name? What is that? It isn't me. It isn't me that gets me up this hill each morning, but rather an irrepressibility that must be called life, life itself, a force working independently of my brain, body and mind. I don't know what it is.

I hoist myself up to sit on the trig point and look out over the city. I know and have walked every inch of that city. What is it that is leaning forward in me now, towards the world? There is a prayer flag tied to the branches of a tree just below me, like the prayer flag I have at home.

What is it that dares to want to get back down this hill and go home and write? Or that wants to find out why things in nature are rarely blue. What is it that triggers the synapses that call to the muscles to work the body and keep going on? What is it that still insists on being happy? What is it that refuses the call of defeat?

∞

Cure for insomnia:

Take a river, lake, ocean or other body of open water; a swimming pool will do if cold enough and outside. Fresh air is key; cold is key. Get in regardless and in any attire, unattired will do if privacy or not-caring allows. Get in. Jumping or diving is best but any approach suffices if the end result is in and so long as head is submerged soon and completely.

Swim against, against, against. Swim into the waves or current if there are waves or current. Thus allowing the body of water to assert itself over your own body and to overwhelm the thinking mind, for it is the thinking mind that is so foregone with thought that it forgets there are things in the world which exist thoughtlessly. Be as often submerged in the thoughtless water as possible. If the river is the Avon, the Frome, the Wye, the

Tarn, the Lot, the Aveyron, take time to look around at the thoughtless landscape: the banks, meadows, willows, boulders, limestone gorge, sandy river-beach, granite outcrop, conifered hillside. This is the present world and excludes all others. If a thought should emerge that is otherwise or otherwhere, head under, drown it.

Swim with, with, with. Swim as the waves or currents go, if there are waves or currents. Thus allowing the body of water to assert itself as an upward and outward force, for it is the downward and inward nature of the thinking mind that brings on the recursions and iterations of sadness and madness. In this English or French river, or this little Wiltshire lake, or this great Atlantic, look about at the spacious air, noting that there is more space than there are things in space, and that the space gives no resistance or argument to anything in it. Nor does the light arbitrate between which things it should fall on and which things not. The light falls and space unfolds. If a thought should emerge that is overly small or turning inward, head under, drown it.

The principle applies for the lake or pool, for when you kick and pull your arms in breaststroke or crawl, know the pushing back of the water in your hands and be aware that the water, even without tide or current, is working against you and braiding backwards. Feel the slight drag. Then, with the forward stroke, know that the water is rushing ahead of your hands. Feel the slight forwards lurch. For there is wisdom in knowing that we are sometimes the cause and influencer of our own currents and tides, which we make in otherwise still waters.

In the lake feel the earthy softness of the water, and in the pool feel the bleached crispness, and in the lake see underwater how your hands emerge as ghost hands in the mill of the stroke, only to evaporate when the stroke recedes, while in the pool your hands are shocks of electric white which trail with the diamonds of sunlit bubbles. To the thinking mind, which sinks its anchor in the past and future where no anchor will fix, tell this: no things are fixed. Even your hands from day to day are not the same hands.

This is the cure for insomnia: no things are fixed. Everything passes, this too. One day, when you're done with it, it will lose its footing and fall away, and you'll drop each night into sleep without knowing how you once found it impossible.

∞

A dream of a huge wave. Standing with my mother at the sea shore and a wave comes, and before we know it it's the size of two houses on top of each other, so we cling on to one another's arms and I open my mouth but no sound comes out.

The wave arcs over us, and as it does its inner surfaces turn into metal panels, so that we are now effectively in a huge domed room which creaks under the weight of water, like a submarine. Its great rolling barrel shifts over us. When it passes we walk out the other side, dry, into open air.

penguin.co.uk/vintage